SECOND EDITION

THE POCKET MANUAL of

OMT

OSTEOPATHIC
MANIPULATIVE
TREATMENT FOR
PHYSICIANS

T0257418

SECOND EDITION

THE POCKET MANUAL of

OMT

OSTEOPATHIC
MANIPULATIVE
TREATMENT FOR
PHYSICIANS

Editor, Co-Author

David R. Beatty, DO

Professor, Osteopathic Principles and Practice
West Virginia School of Osteopathic Medicine
Lewisburg, West Virginia

Co-Author

To Shan Li, DO
Assistant Professor, Osteopathic
 Principles and Practice
West Virginia School of Osteopathic
 Medicine
Lewisburg, West Virginia

Co-Author

Karen M. Steele, DO, FAAO
Professor, Osteopathic Principles and
 Practice
Associate Dean for Osteopathic
 Medical Education
West Virginia School of Osteopathic
 Medicine
Lewisburg, West Virginia

Co-Author

Zachary J. Comeaux, DO, FAAO
Professor, Osteopathic Principles and
 Practice
West Virginia School of Osteopathic
 Medicine
Lewisburg, West Virginia

Co-Author

John M. Garlitz, DO
Assistant Professor, Osteopathic
 Principles and Practice
West Virginia School of Osteopathic
 Medicine
Lewisburg, West Virginia

Co-Author

James W. Kribs, DO
Assistant Professor and Chairperson,
 Osteopathic Principles and Practice
West Virginia School of Osteopathic
 Medicine
Lewisburg, West Virginia

Co-Author

William W. Lemley, DO, FAAO
Professor, Osteopathic Principles and
 Practice
West Virginia School of Osteopathic
 Medicine
Lewisburg, West Virginia

Wolters Kluwer | Lippincott Williams & Wilkins
Health

Philadelphia · Baltimore · New York · London
Buenos Aires · Hong Kong · Sydney · Tokyo

Acquisitions Editor: Charles W. Mitchell
Product Manager: Jennifer Verbiar
Senior Designer: Joan Wendt
Cover Designer: Larry Didona
Compositor: MPS Limited, A Macmillan Company

Second Edition

Library of Congress Cataloging-in-Publication Data

The pocket manual of OMT: osteopathic manipulative treatment for physicians/editor, co-author, David R. Beatty ... [et al.].—2nd ed.
     p.; cm.
     Other title: Osteopathic manipulative treatment for physicians
     Includes bibliographical references and index.
     ISBN 978-1-60831-657-1
     1. Osteopathic medicine—Handbooks, manuals, etc. 2. Osteopathic orthopedics—Handbooks, manuals, etc. 3. Primary care (Medicine)—Handbooks, manuals, etc.
     I. Essig-Beatty, David R. II. Title: Osteopathic manipulative treatment for physicians.
     [DNLM: 1. Manipulation, Osteopathic—methods—Handbooks. 2. Primary Health Care—Handbooks. WB 39 P7393 2011]
     RZ342.P63 2011
     615.5'33—dc22

                                                                                          2010002032

DISCLAIMER

CONTENTS

ACKNOWLEDGMENTS

Thanks are extended to WVSOM graduate teaching assistants Derek Stone for editing and Karl Speers for adaptation of sacral graphics with permission of Kenneth E. Graham, DO. WVSOM students Mark Cabrera, Aaron Kelley, Donald N. Pyle II, Dana Quarles, and Linda Wilson contributed to photography and editing. Karen Ayers of the WVSOM Department of Media Services assisted with photography. William A. Kuchera, DO, FAAO provided his unique drawings of biomechanics through a contract with Dr Beatty for the book *Manipulation at Home: Exercises Based on Osteopathic Structural Exam* (WVSOM, Lewisburg, 2003). Gratitude is extended to Karen Snider, DO who contributed to the development of this book while a graduate teaching assistant at WVSOM through her initial concept and editing of the *Mini-Manual of Muscle Energy and HVLA Techniques* (WVSOM, Lewisburg, 2000) from which this book has evolved.

REVIEWERS

Jane E. Carreiro, DO
Associate Professor
University of New England College of Osteopathic Medicine
Department of Osteopathic Manipulative Medicine
Biddeford, Maine

John C. Glover, DO, FAAO
Chairman, Osteopathic Manipulative Medicine
Touro University, California College of Osteopathic Medicine
Vallejo, California

Kenneth E. Graham, DO
Clinical Associate Professor
Director of Hospital Care for Center for Structural Medicine
Oklahoma State University College of Osteopathic Medicine
Tulsa, Oklahoma

William A. Kuchera, DO, FAAO
Professor Emeritus
Kirksville College of Osteopathic Medicine
Kirksville, Missouri

Kenneth E. Nelson, DO, FAAO
Chicago College of Osteopathic Medicine
Midwestern University
Downers Grove, Illinois

PREFACE

We are pleased to be invited by Lippincott Williams & Wilkins to publish a second edition of *The Pocket Manual of OMT*. The book remains a concise clinical reference for physicians and osteopathic medical students but has many new features based on their feedback. Forty-three new techniques have been added since the first edition as a result of faculty innovation and new recommendations from the Educational Council on Osteopathic Principles of the American Association of Colleges of Osteopathic Medicine. Spiral binding allows the manual to remain open on the treatment table while learning new techniques or treating patients. Updated and expanded descriptions of osteopathic principles and definitions are complemented by additional illustrations and new clinical correlations. Each chapter is supplemented by online case-study questions as well as technique videos at http://thePoint.lww.com. Exercise techniques have been moved from the end of each chapter to immediately following their analogous treatments to facilitate logical prescribing. Lastly, two new techniques, seated facet release and inherent motion diagnosis and treatment, join facilitated oscillatory release[1,2] and percussion vibrator as techniques first published in *The Pocket Manual of OMT*.

Seated facet release technique is an approach to treatment of the vertebral column and ribs in which all diagnosis and treatment occurs with the patient seated and the practitioner standing or seated behind the patient. Each facet joint capsule is palpated during gentle compression and spontaneous recoil. A facet found to be closed or open is treated by positioning the patient so that the facet is at its greatest point of tension, then inducing a gentle compressive or distraction force into that joint. For the cervical, upper thoracic, and rib areas the patient rests against the practitioner's abdomen in order to engage the facet at its greatest point of tension. This technique was taught to one of the authors (KMS) by Richard H. Still, Jr, DO, great grandson of Andrew T. Still, MD, DO, founder of the osteopathic profession. Techniques are shown for treatment of the cervical spine (including the occipitoatlantal joint), first rib, typical ribs, thoracic spine, lumbar spine, and sacroiliac joint.

Inherent motion refers to a cyclic pressure fluctuation palpable anywhere on the body but first identified on the cranium and sacrum by William Garner Sutherland, DO and termed the primary respiratory mechanism. This pressure fluctuation is directly related to cerebrospinal fluid pressure and volume[3,4] and corresponds to pulse pressure fluctuations (Traube–Hering–Mayer waves)[5]. Like any other motion of the body, inherent motion can be assessed for restriction of related tissues and

---

[1]Comeaux ZC. Facilitated oscillatory release—a method of dynamic assessment and treatment of somatic dysfunction. *Am Acad Osteopath J*. 2003;13(3):30–35.

[2]Comeaux ZC. *Harmonic Healing: A Guide to Facilitated Oscillatory Release and Other Rhythmic Myofascial Techniques*. Berkeley, CA: North Atlantic Books; 2008.

[3]Adams T, Heisy RS, Smith MC, et al. Parietal bone mobility in the anesthetized cat. *J Am Osteopath Assoc*. 1992;92(5):599–621.

[4]Heisy SR, Adams T. Role of cranial bone mobility in cranial compliance. *Neurosurgery*. 1993;33(5):869–877.

[5]Nelson KE, Sergueff N, Lipinski CM, et al. Cranial rhythmic impulse related to the Traube–Herring–Mayer oscillation: comparing laser Doppler flowmetry and palpation. *J Am Osteopath Assoc*. 2001;101(3):163–173.

treated using principles of OMT. Techniques for diagnosis and treatment using inherent motion are presented for the lower extremities, pelvis, sacrum, thoracic spine and ribs, and thoracic inlet.

The Pocket Manual of OMT reflects the hard work and critical thinking of the Department of Osteopathic Principles and Practice (OPP) at the West Virginia School of Osteopathic Medicine (WVSOM), a top rated school for primary care and rural medicine. Over the past 20 years we have retained and refined skills important for primary care osteopathic physicians, dropping those techniques that are impractical or overly specialized. This approach to technique selection makes the book useful as both an initial learning tool for students and a practical reference for clinicians.

The Pocket Manual of OMT: Use it to learn osteopathic diagnosis and treatment; keep it handy for clinical applications; copy the exercises for patients. Our goal for this book is the same as that of the first school of osteopathic medicine:

> *To improve our present systems of surgery, obstetrics, and treatment of disease generally, to place the same on a more rational and scientific basis, to impart information to the medical profession . . .*[6]

We hope you will find this manual helpful in providing osteopathic care to your patients. As you choose and apply the techniques, we encourage you to think about the logic behind their use and to adapt them to best suit your patients' needs. We welcome your input as this manual continues to evolve.

David R. Beatty, DO, Editor
To Shan Li, DO
Karen M. Steele, DO, FAAO
Zachary J. Comeaux, DO, FAAO
John M. Garlitz, DO
James W. Kribs, DO
William W. Lemley, DO, FAAO

---

[6]Still AT. *American School of Osteopathy*. Revised Charter. Kirksville, MO: Still National Osteopathic Museum; 1894.

1 Introduction to Osteopathic Diagnosis and Treatment

Osteopathic manipulative treatment (OMT) is used to treat a patient's problem associated with *somatic dysfunction*: impaired or altered function of related components of the somatic (body framework) system—skeletal, arthrodial, and myofascial structures, and related vascular, lymphatic, and neural elements.[1]

Diagnosis of somatic dysfunction is derived from structural examination to identify at least one of four diagnostic criteria described by the mnemonic TART (tissue texture abnormality, asymmetry, restriction of motion, and tenderness). Somatic dysfunction can be described as position of a body part, direction of free motion, or direction of restricted motion. For example, limited ankle dorsiflexion after a sprained ankle could be termed an anterior talus, ankle plantar flexion, or restricted ankle dorsiflexion. Each of these terms describes ankle somatic dysfunction. *The Pocket Manual of OMT* utilizes *restricted motion* terminology when relevant because it is more readily understood by practitioners other than osteopathic physicians.

Structural examination consists of screening the body to identify a region with somatic dysfunction, scanning to identify its location within the region, and local diagnosis to precisely define the somatic dysfunction. Screening tests, including postural exam and gait analysis to identify regional asymmetry, are presented in Chapter 2. Scanning tests and diagnosis skills are presented in subsequent chapters covering the 10 regions of somatic dysfunction: lower extremity, pelvis, sacrum, lumbar, thoracic, rib, upper extremity, cervical, head, and abdominal/other (visceral).

INDICATIONS FOR OMT: Osteopathic manipulative treatment is defined as the therapeutic application of manually guided forces by an osteopathic physician (U.S. usage) to improve physiologic function and/or support homeostasis that have been altered by somatic dysfunction.[1] OMT is indicated whenever the practitioner makes the diagnosis of somatic dysfunction and relates it to a patient's problem. Systematic reviews have demonstrated efficacy of manipulation, in general, for back pain, neck pain, and headache.[2-9] Other conditions amenable to OMT are supported by

CLINICAL CORRELATION: A 25-year-old female osteopathic medical student has had lower back pain for 1 week since playing intramural flag football. She has muscle spasm in the right lumbar erector spinae muscles and tenderness on the right L2–5 transverse processes, which are resistant to anterior pressure compared to the left side. ASSESSMENT: (1) Lumbar strain and sprain; (2) lumbar somatic dysfunction (consisting of L2–5 restricted rotation left).

The lumbar somatic dysfunction could also be described as posterior right L2–5 tender points, right lumbar erector spinae muscle spasm, or L2–5 rotated right. In this case, however, L2–5 restricted rotation left is the most specific description and conveys the functional significance of the findings to nonosteopathic practitioners.

1

small studies or clinical observation and are listed for each technique in subsequent chapters.

CONTRAINDICATIONS TO OMT: The only absolute contraindications to all OMT are absence of somatic dysfunction and patient's desire not to have treatment. An individual technique is contraindicated when its potential benefit is outweighed by the risk of harm to the patient. Indirect techniques in which the body is moved away from a restriction and into a position of tissue laxity incur less risk for patients with acute injuries, severe illnesses, undiagnosed problems, or fragile conditions. Direct techniques in which the body is moved into a restriction are less applicable under these circumstances but are effective and safe for most chronic conditions. Relative contraindications are technique specific and are listed for each treatment presented in subsequent chapters.

OMT TECHNIQUES: Each type of manipulative treatment has principles of application that can be applied to any part of the body based on practitioner knowledge of anatomy and function.

INDIRECT TECHNIQUES (move body into position of laxity to facilitate neurological resetting and local tissue relaxation)

Counterstrain: A system of diagnosis and treatment developed by Lawrence H. Jones, DO, which considers the dysfunction to be a continuing, inappropriate strain reflex that is inhibited by applying a position of mild strain in the direction exactly opposite to that of the reflex. This is accomplished by specific directed positioning about the point of tenderness to achieve the desired therapeutic response.[1]

1. Identify and label tender point as 10/10 or 100%;
2. Passively position the body into tissue laxity and retest for tenderness, fine tuning in all planes of motion until tenderness is minimized to 0/10 if possible but at most 3/10;
3. Hold this position of maximum relief for 90 seconds (120 seconds for ribs), maintaining finger contact to monitor for tissue texture changes but reducing pressure;
4. Slowly and passively return the body to neutral;
5. Retest for tenderness with the same pressure as initial labeling and retreat if not improved.

Facilitated Positional Release: A system of indirect myofascial release treatment developed by Stanley Schiowitz, DO. The component region of the body is placed into a neutral position, diminishing tissue and joint tension in all planes, and an activating force (compression or torsion) is added.[1]

1. Identify tension related to restricted motion;
2. Place the joint or region in its neutral position;
3. Palpate the tension and move the joint or region into its position of laxity for all planes;
4. Add compression or torsion to facilitate tissue laxity;
5. Hold the position of laxity for 3–5 seconds until tension release is completed and then slowly return to neutral;
6. Retest for tension or motion.

Ligamentous Articular Strain: A manipulative technique described by Howard Lippincott, DO and Rebecca Lippincott, DO in which the goal of treatment is to balance the tension in opposing ligaments where abnormal tension is present.[1]

1. Identify ligament or myofascial tension;
2. Press into or apply traction to the tense area to engage the tissues;
3. Slowly move the part of the body into its position of laxity for all planes;
4. Maintain the position of laxity using balanced pressure and follow any tissue release until completed or inherent motion (cranial rhythmic impulse) is palpated;
5. Retest for tension.

DIRECT TECHNIQUES (move body into restriction to facilitate improved motion)

Muscle Energy: A form of osteopathic manipulative diagnosis and treatment developed by Fred Mitchell Sr, DO in which the patient's muscles are actively used on request, from a precisely controlled position, in a specific direction, and against a distinctly executed physician counterforce.[1]

1. Identify restricted joint movement for all possible planes of motion;
2. Move the joint into its restriction for all planes;
3. Have the patient push away from the restriction against equal physician resistance for 3–5 seconds;
4. Allow full relaxation and then slowly move the joint to a new restrictive barrier;
5. Repeat isometric contraction and stretch 3–5 times;
6. Retest motion.

Soft Tissue: A direct technique that usually involves lateral stretching, linear stretching, deep pressure, traction, and/or separation of muscle origin and insertion while monitoring tissue response and motion changes by palpation.[1]

1. Identify tension or edema;
2. Apply force to the tense or edematous tissues by:
   a. Longitudinal stretch (traction);
   b. Kneading (lateral stretch);
   c. Inhibition (sustained pressure);
   d. Effleurage (stroking pressure);
   e. Petrissage (squeezing pressure);
3. Retest for tension or edema.

Thrust: An osteopathic technique employing a rapid, therapeutic force of brief duration that travels a short distance within the anatomic range of motion of a joint, and that engages the restrictive barrier in one or more planes of motion to elicit release of restriction. Also known as high velocity low amplitude (HVLA).[1]

1. Identify restricted joint movement for all possible planes of motion;
2. Move the joint into its restriction for all planes;
3. Apply a short quick thrust through one of the restricted joint planes;
4. Retest motion.

COMBINED TECHNIQUES (use both indirect and direct mechanisms)

Articulatory: A low velocity/moderate-to-high amplitude technique in which a joint is carried through its full motion, with the therapeutic goal of increased freedom of range of movement. The activating force is either a repetitive springing motion or repetitive concentric movement of the joint through the restrictive barrier.[1]

1. Identify restricted joint movement for all possible planes of motion;
2. Slowly move the joint to its position of laxity for all planes;
3. Slowly move the joint into its restriction for all planes;
4. Repeat as one smooth movement 3–5 times until joint mobility returns;
5. Retest motion.

Facilitated Oscillatory Release: A manipulative technique developed by Zachary J. Comeaux, DO that applies manual oscillatory force to normalize neuromuscular function, intended to be combined with any treatment involving ligamentous or myofascial techniques.[10,11]

1. Identify tension and asymmetry related to restricted motion;
2. Initiate stretch and oscillatory motion of the region of restriction using some tissue mass to initiate a standing (harmonic) wave;
3. Monitor the quality of motion response in the tissues to further localize restriction;
4. Continue rhythmic oscillation or modify its force until tension is reduced or rhythmic mobility improves. Other corrective force may be combined;
5. Retest for tension or motion restriction.

Myofascial Release: A system of diagnosis and treatment first described by Andrew T. Still and his early students that engages continual palpatory feedback to achieve release of myofascial tissues.[1]

1. Identify restricted tissue or joint movement for all possible planes of motion;
2. Indirect: Slowly move the part of the body into its position of laxity for all planes and follow any tissue release until completed;
3. Direct: Slowly move the part of the body into its restrictions for all planes and apply steady force until tissue give is completed;
4. Retest motion.

Osteopathy in the Cranial Field (cranial): A system of diagnosis and treatment first described by William G. Sutherland, DO and applied by an osteopathic practitioner using the primary respiratory mechanism and balanced membranous tension.[1]

Primary Respiratory Mechanism: A conceptual model that describes a process involving five interactive, involuntary functions: (1) The inherent motility of the brain and spinal cord, (2) fluctuation of the cerebrospinal fluid, (3) mobility of the intracranial and intraspinal membranes, (4) articular mobility of the cranial bones, and (5) mobility of the sacrum between the ilia (pelvic bones) that is interdependent with the motion at the sphenobasilar synchondrosis.[1]

Seated Facet Release: A system of diagnosis and treatment taught to one of the authors (KMS) by Richard H. Still Jr, DO, great-grandson of Andrew T. Still, MD, DO, in which the patient is seated and the practitioner stands or sits behind him or her. The patient is guided into the position of greatest tension for a restricted open or closed facet. Then compression or distraction is introduced to that individual facet causing release of the restriction.

1. Stand or sit behind the seated patient;
2. Let the patient increase lordosis or kyphosis to balance the shoulders over the pelvis for lower spine and sacroiliac areas, or lean against you for upper spine and rib areas;

3. Place a knuckle or finger on the inferior facet of the locked open or locked closed facet group;
4. Place your other hand on the shoulder or head and gently compress inferiorly while extending the involved spinal or rib region, keeping the shoulders balanced over the pelvis for lower spine and sacroiliac areas or the patient leaning against you for upper spine and rib areas;
5. Test for the position of greatest restriction by gentle compression and recoil to close and open the locked facet;
6. Hold the patient in the position of greatest restriction and gently apply a small amount of additional compression or traction to induce glide of the facet, thereby releasing the restriction;
7. Retest motion.

Visceral: A system of diagnosis and treatment directed to the viscera to improve physiologic function; typically the viscera are moved toward their fascial attachments to a point of fascial balance; also called ventral techniques.[1]

OTHER TECHNIQUES (do not use barrier concept as a treatment principle)

Lymphatic Pump: A term used to describe the impact of intrathoracic pressure changes on lymphatic flow. This was the name originally given to the thoracic pump technique before the more extensive physiologic effects of the technique were recognized.[1]

Percussion Vibrator: A manipulative technique developed by Robert Fulford, DO involving the specific application of mechanical vibratory force to treat somatic dysfunction.[1]

1. Identify tension or restricted movement;
2. Place the percussion pad on an associated bony prominence with the pad oriented perpendicular to the surface;
3. Alter pad speed, pressure, and angle until vibrations are palpated as strong by a monitoring hand placed on the opposite side of the tension or restriction;
4. Maintain contact until the force and rhythm of vibrations return to that of normal tissue;
5. Alternate technique:
   a. Allow the monitoring hand to be pulled toward the pad, resisting any other direction of pull;
   b. Maintain percussion until the monitoring hand is pushed away from the pad;
6. Slowly release the monitoring hand and percussor pad and retest for tension or restriction.

Somatovisceral Reflexes: A localized somatic stimulation producing patterns of reflex response in segmentally related visceral structures.[1] Treatment techniques for sympathetic normalization include rib raising, thoracolumbar inhibition, abdominal plexus release, Chapman point stimulation, and treatment of thoracolumbar-facilitated segments. Techniques for parasympathetic normalization include suboccipital inhibition or other occipitoatlantal treatments and sacral rocking or other sacroiliac treatments.

EXERCISE TECHNIQUES: Exercises derived from structural exam and OMT are presented after their corresponding treatment techniques.[12] Type of exercise prescribed depends on the patient assessment, somatic dysfunction present, contraindications present, and response to OMT.

CLINICAL CORRELATION: A 25-year-old female osteopathic medical student has had lower back pain for 1 week since playing intramural flag football. She has muscle spasm in the right lumbar erector spinae muscles and tenderness on the right L2–5 transverse processes, which are resistant to anterior pressure compared to the left side. ASSESSMENT: (1) Lumbar strain and sprain; (2) lumbar somatic dysfunction. **PLAN: OMT to lumbar region using counterstrain and indirect myofascial release resulting in reduced tenderness and tension and improved motion.**

Since this is a case of acute strain and sprain, the indirect techniques of counterstrain and myofascial release were applied. In the case of incomplete resolution of the restriction with these treatments, direct techniques such as muscle energy or thrust could be applied but with a risk for symptom exacerbation or worsening of an acute sprain. No evidence of inflammation (swelling, redness, and heat) or neurological involvement and patient tolerance of the restrictive barrier would favor applying direct techniques on the first visit.

Position of Ease: Resting in a position for shortening of tense tissues for 2–5 minutes to bring about relaxation and decrease pain; useful for myofascial tenderness associated with acute problems as well as pain relief for subacute and chronic problems; contraindicated for acute fractures.

Stretching: A steady movement into a restriction for 10–20 seconds to reduce tension and restore motion; useful for tension associated with subacute and chronic problems; contraindicated for acute sprains, acute fractures, or joint instability.

Self-Mobilization: A short and quick or slow and repetitive movement into a restriction to restore joint mobility; useful for joint restrictions associated with subacute and chronic problems; contraindicated for acute sprains, acute fractures, joint instability, inflammation, severe degeneration, or severe osteoporosis.

Postural Strengthening: A contraction of postural muscles against gravitational resistance until fatigued and repeated every other day to restore strength for standing and walking.

PRESCRIBING OMT: Each treatment plan depends upon the patient's preference, physician's skill, history, exam findings, indications, contraindications, and response to treatment. Exercises, orthotics, braces, and thermal therapy can be prescribed to complement the effectiveness of OMT. Cold packs can be applied for 15–20 minutes to inflamed or painful areas to reduce swelling and pain. Hot packs can be applied for 20–30 minutes before or after treatment or exercise to reduce tension, stiffness, and ache. Pain due to hypermobility or ligamentous laxity can be temporarily reduced with indirect methods of manipulation but is better treated with stabilization techniques such as bracing, strengthening, and prolotherapy. The latter, also called sclerotherapy, uses injection of a proliferant solution into weakened ligaments to strengthen or shorten the lax tissues.[13] The prescription of OMT is an art in which the physician uses structural diagnosis and appropriate treatment to improve patient's functioning so that healing may occur more readily.

CLINICAL CORRELATION: A 25-year-old female osteopathic medical student has had lower back pain for 1 week since playing intramural flag football. She has muscle spasm in the right lumbar erector spinae muscles and tenderness on the right L2–5 transverse processes, which are resistant to anterior pressure compared to the left side. ASSESSMENT: (1) Lumbar strain and sprain; (2) lumbar somatic dysfunction. PLAN: (1) OMT to lumbar region using counterstrain and indirect myofascial release resulting in reduced tenderness and tension and improved motion; **(2) cold pack to low back for 15 minutes 3–4 times a day if needed for pain relief; (3) heating pad to low back for 20 minutes 3–4 times a day if needed for stiffness; and (4) lumbar extensor stretches twice a day if tolerated.**

If she failed to improve after 2–3 additional treatments using a variety of techniques over 2 weeks, re-evaluation should be conducted for postural problems, hypermobility, disc and joint problems, and referred pain. Additional treatment options should emerge from this re-evaluation.

REFERENCES

1. Glossary Review Committee. *Glossary of Osteopathic Terminology*. Chevy Chase, MD: Educational Council on Osteopathic Principles of the American Association of Colleges of Osteopathic Medicine; 2009.
2. Bronfort G, Assendelft WJ, Evans R, et al. Efficacy of spinal manipulation for chronic headache: a systematic review. *J Manipulative Physiol Ther*. 2001; 24(7):457–466.
3. Bronfort G, Haas M, Evans R, et al. Efficacy of spinal manipulation and mobilization for low back pain and neck pain: a systematic review and best evidence synthesis. *Spine J*. 2004;4(3):335–356.
4. Gross AR, Hoving JL, Haines TA, et al. A Cochrane review of manipulation and mobilization for mechanical neck disorders. *Spine*. 2004;15(29): 1541–1548.
5. Gross AR, Kay T, Hondras M, et al. Manual therapy for mechanical neck disorders: a systematic review. *Man Ther*. 2002;7(3):131–149.
6. Hurwitz EL, Aker PD, Adams AH, et al. Manipulation and mobilization of the cervical spine: a systematic review of the literature. *Spine*. 1996;21(15): 1746–1759.
7. Koes BW, Assendelft WJ, Van der Heijden G, et al. Spinal manipulation for low back pain: an updated systematic review of randomized clinical trials. *Spine*. 1996;21(24):2860–2871.
8. Pengel HM. Systematic review of conservative interventions for subacute low back pain. *Clin Rehabil*. 2002;16(8):811–820.
9. van Tulder MW, Koes BW, Bouter LM. Conservative treatment of acute and chronic nonspecific low back pain: a systematic review of randomized controlled trials of the most common interventions. *Spine*. 1997;22(18): 2128–2156.
10. Comeaux ZC. Facilitated oscillatory release—a method of dynamic assessment and treatment of somatic dysfunction. *AAO J*. 2003;13(3):30–35.

11. Comeaux ZC. *Harmonic Healing: A Guide to Facilitated Oscillatory Release and Other Rhythmic Myofascial Techniques.* Berkeley, California: North Atlantic Books; 2008.
12. Essig-Beatty DR. *Manipulation at Home: Exercises Based on Osteopathic Structural Examination.* Lewisburg, PA: WVSOM; 2003.
13. Ravin T, Cantieri M, Pasquarello G. *Principles of Prolotherapy.* Denver, CO: American Academy of Musculoskeletal Medicine; 2008.

Postural Diagnosis and Treatment

Diagnosis of Postural Problems:
1. Dynamic postural evaluation *p. 9*
2. Static posture—posterior *p. 10*
3. Static posture—lateral *p. 11*
4. Scoliosis evaluation (if indicated) *p. 12*
5. Short leg evaluation (if indicated) *p. 13*
6. Hypermobility screening *p. 14*

Postural Treatment:
1. Heel lift therapy *p. 16*
2. Spinal flexibility exercises *p. 17*
3. Spinal mobility exercises *p. 17*
4. Postural strengthening exercises *p. 18*

Diagnosis

DYNAMIC POSTURAL EVALUATION

1. Stand behind the barefoot patient and observe walking 5–10 steps away from and then toward you;

2. Identify areas of asymmetrical and decreased movement:

   a) Stride;
   b) Heel strike/toe off;
   c) Lower extremity rotation;
   d) Pelvic levelness and rotation;
   e) Trunk rotation;
   f) Shoulder levelness;
   g) Arm swing;
   h) Head levelness.

3. Common abnormalities:

   a) Asymmetry due to weakness;
   b) Asymmetry due to restriction;
   c) Decreased movement due to restriction;
   d) Neurological disorders: Foot drop, foot slapping, shuffling, wide stanced, staggering, lurching.

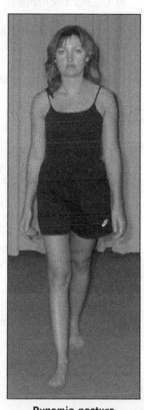

Dynamic posture

9

STATIC POSTURE—POSTERIOR

1. Stand behind the barefoot patient and observe an imaginary vertical line upward from halfway between the medial malleoli;

2. The vertical line should normally pass:

   a) Halfway between the knees;
   b) Along the gluteal fold;
   c) Through all spinous processes;
   d) Along the midline of the head.

3. Observe for horizontal levelness of:

   a) Popliteal creases;
   b) Greater trochanters;
   c) Iliac crests;
   d) Inferior angles of scapula;
   e) Tops of shoulders;
   f) Mastoid processes.

4. Observe for symmetry of:

   a) Foot rotation;
   b) Arm length;
   c) Arm distance from torso.

5. Palpate:

   a) Foot arches by sliding fingertips under the medial arches;
   b) Achilles tendon tension.

6. Common abnormalities:

   a) Foot external rotation;
   b) Pes planus (fallen foot arch);
   c) Iliac crest asymmetry;
   d) Pelvic side shift;
   e) Sacral base unleveling;
   f) Scoliosis;
   g) Shoulder height asymmetry;
   h) Head tilt.

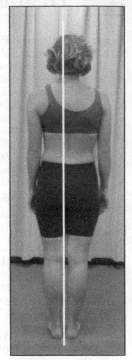

Right pelvic shift

STATIC POSTURE—LATERAL

1. Stand lateral to the barefoot patient and observe an imaginary weight bearing line upward from the anterior aspect of the lateral malleolus;

2. The weight-bearing line should normally pass through:

   a) Anterior aspect of lateral malleolus;
   b) Middle of tibial plateau;
   c) Greater trochanter;
   d) Body of L3 (center of body mass);
   e) Middle of humeral head;
   f) External auditory meatus.

3. Common abnormalities:

   a) Anterior head carriage;
   b) Shoulder anterior or posterior;
   c) Thoracic hyperkyphosis;
   d) Lumbar hyperlordosis;
   e) Anterior pelvic weight bearing.

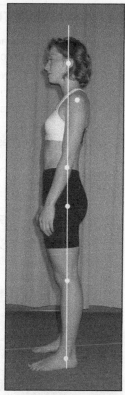

Posterior shoulders

SCOLIOSIS EVALUATION (forward bending or Adam's test)

1. Stand behind the barefoot patient and ask him or her to slowly bend forward and reach for the ground with the legs straight;

2. A rib hump with forward bending indicates possible scoliosis convex to the side of the fullness;

3. If a rib hump is present, ask the patient to bend to the side of fullness;

4. A rib hump that goes away with sidebending to that side indicates a functional scoliosis while one that remains indicates a structural scoliosis.

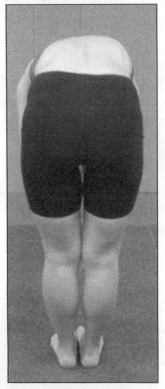

Right rib hump (right scoliosis)

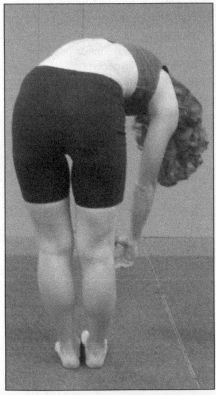

Diminished with sidebending (functional scoliosis)

Short Leg Evaluation

ILIAC CREST HEIGHT

1. Stand behind the barefoot patient;
2. Place your fingertips on the superior surface of the iliac crests in the mid-axillary line;
3. An inferior iliac crest indicates a relative short leg;
4. Common causes of asymmetry:
   a) Pes planus or cavus;
   b) Genu valgum or varus;
   c) Knee or hip restriction;
   d) Pelvic rotation;
   e) Anatomical short leg.

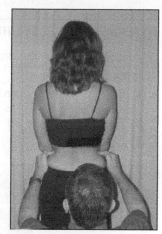

Iliac crest height

MEDIAL MALLEOLUS LEVELNESS

1. Stand at the foot of the supine patient;
2. To seat the pelvis, have the patient bend the knees, lift and set the buttocks down, and straighten out the legs (see *p. 66*);
3. Place your thumbs on the inferior surface of the medial malleoli;
4. With your head centered directly above the ankles, compare your thumbs for superior–inferior levelness of the medial malleoli;

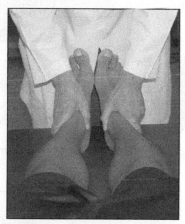

Medial malleolus levelness

5. If medial malleoli are asymmetrical, check ASIS levelness to determine relative leg length;
6. Common causes of asymmetry: knee, hip, or pelvis somatic dysfunction; anatomical short leg.

HYPERMOBILITY SCREENING (nondominant limb)[1]

A score of 4–5/5 indicates probable generalized hypermobility.

1. Index finger extension
   a) Rest the patient's palm on a flat surface and pull the index finger into extension as far as it will comfortably go;
   b) Finger extension to 90° or more = 1 point.

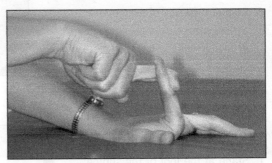

Index finger extension >90°

2. Thumb flexion
   a) Flex the patient's thumb toward the ventral forearm as far as it will comfortably go;
   b) Thumb contact with forearm = 1 point.

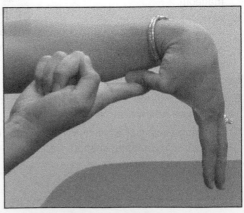

Thumb flexion to ventral forearm

3. Elbow extension
   a) Hold the upper arm with one hand and the wrist with your other hand;
   b) Slowly extend the elbow as far as it will comfortably go;
   c) Elbow extension $\geq 10°$ = 1 point.

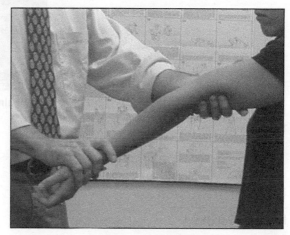

Elbow extension 5°

4. Knee extension
   a) With the patient sitting, hold the thigh with one hand and extend the knee with your other hand as far as it will comfortably go;
   b) Extension $\geq 10°$ = 1 point.

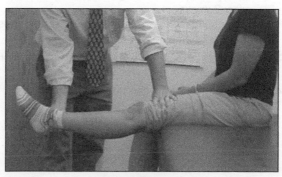

Knee extension 0°

5. Standing flexion

    a) Ask the patient to bend forward as far as is comfortable with the legs straight;

    b) Palms flat on the floor = 1 point.

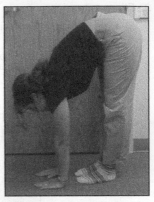

Palms flat on floor

Total Score:

    0/5–3/5: Generalized hypermobility unlikely

    4/5–5/5: Generalized hypermobility likely

Postural Treatment

HEEL LIFT THERAPY

INDICATIONS: Anatomical short leg or sacral base unleveling related to lumbar scoliosis, back pain, and other problems.

PROTOCOL:

1. Perform OMT for lower extremity, pelvis, sacrum, lumbar, and related thoracic, rib, cervical, and head somatic dysfunction;

2. Insert 1/8" heel lift into the shoe on the side of the short leg except for:

    a) Fragile patients (severe pain, radiculopathy, elderly, severe arthritis, severe osteoporosis)—begin with 1/16" lift and increase by 1/16" every 2 weeks;

    b) Recent sudden loss of leg length (fracture, prosthesis)—begin with entire amount of needed lift;

3. Increase lift by 1/8" every 2 weeks as tolerated following OMT until there is iliac crest levelness with standing;

4. Up to 1/2" of heel lift can be used before foot tilt requires that any additional lift be added to the entire sole.

SPINAL FLEXIBILITY EXERCISES

INDICATIONS: Muscle tension related to postural strain, scoliosis, short leg syndrome, back pain, neck pain, headache, stress, anxiety, and other problems.

CONTRAINDICATIONS: Acute strain, sprain, or fracture; hypermobility; undiagnosed radiculopathy; unexplained fever or weight loss.

EXERCISES: Do the following exercises 1–4 times a day if tolerated.

1. Hamstring stretch (*p. 36*)
2. Lumbar extensor stretch (*p. 130*)
3. Thoracolumbar stretch (*p. 117*)
4. Thoracic flexor/extensor stretch (*p. 160*)
5. Cervical extensor stretch (*p. 204*)

SPINAL MOBILITY EXERCISES

INDICATIONS: Restricted motion related to postural strain, scoliosis, short leg syndrome, back pain, neck pain, headache, stress, anxiety, and other problems.

CONTRAINDICATIONS: Acute strain, sprain, or fracture; hypermobility; cancer; joint inflammation; severe joint degeneration; severe osteoporosis; undiagnosed radiculopathy; unexplained fever or weight loss.

EXERCISES: Do the following exercises up to twice a day if tolerated.

1. Sacroiliac self-mobilization (*p. 110*)
2. Lumbar self-mobilization (*p. 134*)
3. Thoracolumbar stretch/self-mobilization (*p. 134*)
4. Thoracic/rib self-mobilization—supine (*p. 163*)
5. Cervical sidebending self-mobilization (*p. 220*)

POSTURAL STRENGTHENING EXERCISES

INDICATIONS: Postural weakness related to inactivity, hypermobility, back pain, neck pain, headache, and other problems.

CONTRAINDICATIONS: Acute strain, sprain, or fracture; unstable cardiac arrhythmia; undiagnosed radiculopathy; unexplained fever or weight loss.

EXERCISES: Do one of the following routines daily or every other day.

Beginner:

1. Pelvic tilt (*p. 18*)
2. Supine leg lift—one leg (*p. 19*)
3. Prone leg lift—one leg (*p. 21*)

Intermediate:

1. Supine leg lift—both legs (*p. 20*)
2. Prone limb lift— one leg and arm (*p. 21*)
3. Abdominal curl (*p. 19*)

Advanced (wrist and ankle weights may be added if needed to reach fatigue by the third repetition):

1. Supine limb lift—both legs and arms (*p. 20*)
2. Prone limb lift—both legs and arms (*p. 22*)

Pelvic Tilt

1. Lie on your back with knees bent and feet flat on the floor;
2. Roll the pelvis back by pushing the low back into the floor and lifting the coccyx (tip of tailbone) slightly upward;
3. Take a few deep breaths and hold this position for 5–20 seconds;
4. Repeat 5–10 times.

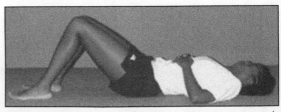

Pelvic tilt

Abdominal Curl

1. Lie on your back with knees bent, feet on the floor, and arms crossed;
2. Slowly lift your head and shoulders until the head is 3–6 inches from the floor;
3. Hold your head and shoulders in this position for 20 seconds;
4. Repeat 3 times;
5. If the third lift is easy, increase the time by 10 seconds.

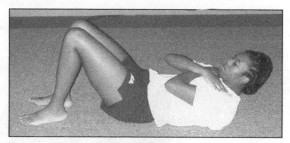

Abdominal curl

Supine Leg Lift—One Leg

1. Lie on your back with one knee bent and that foot on the floor;
2. Allow your bent knee to fall to the side, and slowly lift the entire leg until your foot is 3–6 inches from the floor;
3. Hold your leg in this position for 10 seconds;
4. Repeat for the other leg;
5. Do this leg lift 3 times for each leg. If the third lift is easy, increase the time held by 10 seconds;
6. Do this exercise every other day.

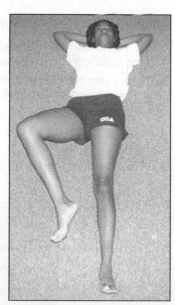

Supine leg lift—one leg

Supine Leg Lift—Both Legs

1. Lie on your back with the legs straight and toes pointing downward;
2. Tighten your buttocks and slowly lift the legs until your feet are 3–6 inches from the floor;
3. Hold your legs in this position for 20 seconds;
4. Repeat this leg lift 3 times. If the third lift is easy, increase the time held by 10 seconds;
5. Do this exercise every other day.

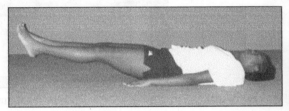

Supine leg lift—both legs

Supine Limb Lift—Legs and Arms

1. Lie on your back with the legs straight, toes pointing downward, and arms straightened above your head;
2. Tighten your buttocks and slowly lift the legs, arms, and head until your hands and feet are 3–6 inches from the floor;
3. Hold your legs, arms, and head in this position for 30 seconds;
4. Repeat 3 times. If the third lift is easy, increase the time held by 10 seconds;
5. Do this exercise every other day.

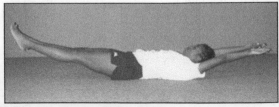

Supine limb lift—legs and arms

Prone Leg Lift—One Leg

1. Lie on your stomach with the legs straight and toes pointing downward;
2. Slowly lift one leg until your foot is 3–6 inches from the floor;
3. Hold your leg in this position for 10 seconds;
4. Repeat 3 times. If the third lift is easy, increase the time held by 10 seconds;
5. Do this exercise every other day.

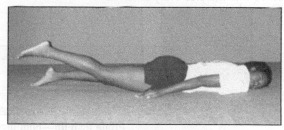

Prone leg lift—one leg

Prone Limb Lift—One Leg and Arm

1. Lie on your stomach with the legs straight, toes pointing downward, and arms straightened above your head;
2. Slowly lift one leg and the opposite arm until your foot and hand are 3–6 inches from the floor;
3. Hold your leg and arm in this position for 20 seconds;
4. Repeat 3 times. If the third lift is easy, increase the time held by 10 seconds;
5. Do this exercise every other day.

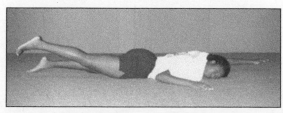

Prone limb lift—one leg and arm

Prone Limb Lift—Both Legs and Arms

1. Lie on your stomach with the legs straight, toes pointing downward, and arms straightened above your head;

2. Push your pubic bone onto the floor and slowly lift both legs, both arms, and your head until the feet and hands are 3–6 inches from the floor;

3. Hold your legs and arms in this position for 30 seconds;

4. Repeat 3 times. If the third lift is easy, increase the time held by 10 seconds;

5. Do this exercise every other day.

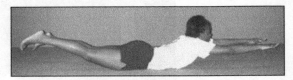

Prone limb lift—both legs and arms

REFERENCE

1. Acasuso-Diaz M, Cisnal A, Collantes-Estevez E. Quantification of joint laxity: the non-dominant (Spanish) modification (letter). *Br J Rheumatol*. 1995;34: 795–796.

3 Lower Extremity Diagnosis and Treatment

Diagnosis of Lower Extremity Somatic Dysfunction:
1. Lower extremity screening *p. 24*
2. Lower extremity palpation *p. 26*
3. Hip range of motion *p. 27*
4. Lower extremity somatic dysfunction diagnosis (Table 3-1) *p. 28*

Treatment of Lower Extremity Somatic Dysfunction:
1. OMT
   Lower extremity facilitated oscillatory release *p. 29*
   Lateral trochanter counterstrain *p. 30*
   Hip myofascial release *p. 31*
   Hip myofascial release—long lever *p. 32*
   Hip/pelvis percussion vibrator *p. 33*
   Hip muscle energy *p. 34*
   Knee motion testing *p. 37*
   Tibial torsion palpation *p. 38*
   Drawer test *p. 38*
   Patella tendon counterstrain *p. 39*
   Meniscus counterstrain *p. 40*
   Anterior cruciate counterstrain *p. 41*
   Posterior cruciate counterstrain *p. 42*
   Knee myofascial release *p. 43*
   Knee percussion vibrator *p. 44*
   Knee articulatory *p. 45*
   Anterior tibia thrust *p. 46*
   Posterior tibia thrust *p. 47*
   Ankle motion *p. 47*
   Ankle swing test *p. 48*
   Extension ankle counterstrain *p. 48*
   Lateral ankle counterstrain *p. 49*
   Medial ankle counterstrain *p. 50*
   Ankle myofascial release *p. 51*
   Ankle muscle energy *p. 52*
   Ankle thrust *p. 53*
   Interosseous membrane myofascial release *p. 54*
   Fibular head motion *p. 55*
   Fibular head muscle energy *p. 55*
   Anterior fibular head thrust *p. 56*
   Posterior fibular head thrust *p. 57*
   Calcaneus counterstrain *p. 59*
   Forefoot myofascial release *p. 60*
   Foot articulatory *p. 60*
   Tarsal thrust *p. 61*
   Interphalangeal articulatory *p. 61*

2. Exercises
    Hip abductor position of ease *p. 32*
    Hamstring stretch *p. 36*
    Hip abductor stretch *p. 36*
    Patella position of ease *p. 40*
    Medial meniscus position of ease *p. 41*
    Hamstring position of ease *p. 44*
    Patella self-mobilization *p. 46*
    Achilles/gastrocnemius position of ease *p. 49*
    Lateral ankle position of ease *p. 50*
    Achilles/gastrocnemius stretch *p. 52*

Diagnosis

Lower Extremity Screening

1. With the patient supine, grasp the feet and test external and internal rotation, comparing sides to identify a restriction;
        If restricted, evaluate knee and hip motion.

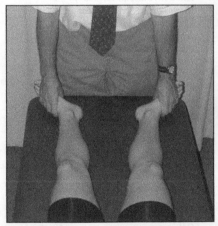

Lower extremity rotation screening

Hip Joint Screening (FABERE test, Patrick maneuver)

1. With the patient supine, passively flex the hip and knee to 90°;

2. Holding the knee with one hand and the ankle with the other, abduct and externally rotate the hip to its restrictive barriers;

3. Maintain the abduction and external rotation barriers as you extend the leg fully;

4. Compare with the other hip to determine restricted motion;

5. Reproduction of hip or pelvic pain suggests hip joint or sacroiliac arthralgia.

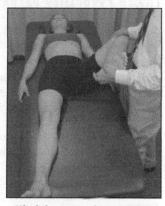

Hip joint screening (FABERE test, Patrick maneuver)

Lower Extremity Diagnosis Using Inherent Motion*

1. With the patient supine, sit or stand comfortably at the foot of the table and place your hands gently over the lower legs;

2. Palpate inherent external and internal rotation;

3. Restricted bilateral external rotation indicates inherent flexion restriction;

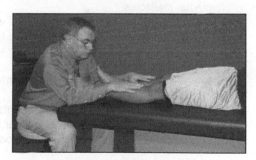

Palpation of inherent motion of the lower extremities

4. Restricted unilateral external rotation indicates lower extremity or pelvis external rotation restriction on the same side;

5. Restricted bilateral internal rotation indicates inherent extension restriction;

6. Restricted unilateral internal rotation indicates lower extremity or pelvis internal rotation restriction on the same side.

---

*The term *inherent motion* refers to a palpable cyclic pressure fluctuation variably referred to as cranial rhythmic impulse, craniosacral motion, entrainment, primary respiratory mechanism, pulse pressure fluctuation, and Traube–Hering–Mayer wave.

LOWER EXTREMITY PALPATION

1. Palpate the lower extremity for tenderness, tension, and edema at the following locations:

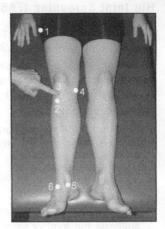
Lower extremity anteromedial palpation

1. Greater trochanter—**lateral trochanter tender point** can be on the trochanter or inferior to it in the iliotibial band;
2. Tibial tuberosity—inferior to patella;
3. **Patella tendon tender point**—superior to tibial tuberosity and inferior to patella;
4. **Medial meniscus tender point**—on tibial plateau medial to middle of patella;
   Cruciate tender point—anterior cruciate in distal medial hamstring, posterior cruciate in popliteus muscle near posterior tibial plateau;
5. **Medial ankle tender point**—ligaments inferior and anterior to medial malleolus;
6. Metatarsal heads—dorsal foot at distal arch;
7. Fibular head—inferior and posterior to lateral knee joint;
8. **Extension ankle tender point**—medial or lateral insertion of gastrocnemius muscle;
9. **Lateral ankle tender point**—ligaments inferior and anterior to lateral malleolus;
10. **Calcaneus tender point**—inferior and anterior aspect of heel;
11. Navicular bone—medial side of plantar foot distal to calcaneus;
12. Cuboid bone—lateral side of plantar foot distal to calcaneus.

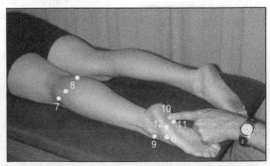
**Lower extremity posterolateral palpation
(cruciate tender points not shown)**

HIP RANGE OF MOTION

With the patient supine, test hip range of motion for each plane of the involved hip and compare with the other side.

1. Abduction—grasp the ankle and move the leg laterally to the abduction barrier;

2. Adduction—grasp the ankle and move the leg medially over the other leg to the adduction barrier;

3. Flexion—palpate the opposite anterior superior iliac spine (ASIS) with one hand, grasp the ankle with the other, and lift the straightened leg to the flexion barrier, which occurs when the opposite ASIS starts to move;

4. Extension— have the patient pull the opposite knee toward the chest and allow the involved leg to hang off the table into the extension barrier, which should normally have the thigh resting on the table;

5. External rotation—flex the hip and knee 90°, hold the knee and ankle, and move the knee laterally to the external rotation barrier;

6. Internal rotation—flex the hip and knee 90°, hold the knee and ankle, and move the knee medially to the internal rotation barrier.

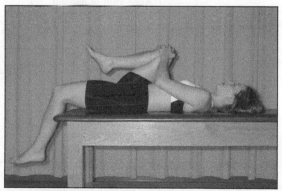

Restricted left hip extension (Thomas test)

Table 3-1 | LOWER EXTREMITY SOMATIC DYSFUNCTION DIAGNOSIS

Somatic Dysfunction[1a] (position of laxity)	Palpatory Findings	Restriction
Metatarsal inferior glide	Tarsal–metatarsal tenderness	Metatarsal superior glide
Metatarsal superior glide	Tarsal–metatarsal tenderness	Metatarsal inferior glide
Navicular inversion	Flat foot Navicular tenderness	Navicular eversion
Cuboid inversion	Flat foot Cuboid tenderness	Cuboid eversion
Talus anterior (relative to tibia)	Gastrocnemius tension and tenderness	Ankle dorsiflexion
Talus posterior (relative to tibia)	Tibialis anterior tension and tenderness	Ankle plantar flexion
Fibular head posterior	Fibular head tenderness	Ankle dorsiflexion Fibular head anterolateral glide
Fibular head anterior	Fibular head tenderness	Ankle plantar flexion Fibular head posteromedial glide
Interosseous torsion	Tibialis anterior tension	Interosseous torsion
Tibia anterior	Knee joint tenderness	Knee extension Posterior drawer
Tibia posterior	Knee joint tenderness	Knee flexion Anterior drawer
Tibia external rotation	Tibial tuberosity lateral Knee joint or patellar tendon tenderness	Tibia internal rotation
Tibia internal rotation	Tibial tuberosity medial Knee joint or patellar tendon tenderness	Tibia external rotation
Hip abduction	Greater trochanter or iliotibial band tenderness Gluteus tension or tenderness	Hip adduction
Hip adduction	Hip adductor tension or tenderness	Hip abduction
Hip extension	Hamstring or gluteal tension or tenderness	Hip flexion
Hip flexion	Quadriceps or iliopsoas tension or tenderness	Hip extension
Hip external rotation	Gluteal or piriformis tension or tenderness	Hip internal rotation (posterior glide)
Hip internal rotation	Hip adductor tension or tenderness	Hip external rotation (anterior glide)

[a]Somatic dysfunction is described by direction of freer motion but can also be defined by position of a body part or direction of restricted motion.

28

Treatment

LOWER EXTREMITY FACILITATED OSCILLATORY RELEASE

INDICATIONS: Lower extremity somatic dysfunction associated with back pain, pelvic pain, leg pain, gait abnormality, and other problems.

RELATIVE CONTRAINDICATIONS: Acute fracture, deep venous thrombosis, or significant patient guarding.

TECHNIQUE (supine):

1. Standing at the foot of the table, grasp the ankle with one or both hands and lift the leg;

2. Internally rotate the leg and lean backward to stretch the fascia of the lower extremity, adjusting the vector of traction to localize restriction;

3. Initiate oscillatory motion of the leg in a horizontal plane by rhythmically moving your arms left and right, feeling for restricted mobility;

4. Continue lower extremity oscillation or modify its traction and force until you feel mobility improve.

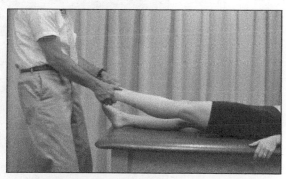

Lower extremity facilitated oscillatory release

LATERAL TROCHANTER COUNTERSTRAIN

INDICATIONS: Lateral trochanter tender point associated with hip pain, back pain, leg pain, gait abnormality, and other problems.

RELATIVE CONTRAINDICATIONS: Deep venous thrombosis.

TECHNIQUE (supine):

1. Hold the ankle with one hand and locate the tender point on the lateral thigh between the greater trochanter and the knee, labeling it 10/10;

2. Abduct and slightly externally rotate the leg and retest for tenderness;

3. Fine-tune this position with slightly more abduction or external rotation until tenderness is minimized to 0/10 if possible, but at most to 3/10;

4. Hold this position for 90 seconds, maintaining finger contact to monitor for tissue texture changes, but reducing pressure;

5. Slowly and passively return the leg to neutral and retest for tenderness, using the same pressure as initial labeling.

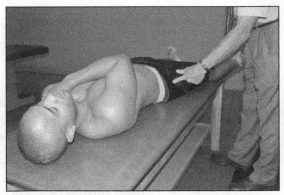

Lateral trochanter counterstrain

HIP MYOFASCIAL RELEASE

INDICATIONS: Restricted hip motion related to hip pain, low back pain, pelvic pain, gait abnormality, and other problems.

RELATIVE CONTRAINDICATIONS: Acute hip fracture or dislocation, deep venous thrombosis, or severe hip or knee osteoarthritis.

TECHNIQUE (supine):

1. Flex the hip and knee to 90° and test internal rotation and external rotation to determine direction of laxity and restriction;

2. Indirect: Move the hip to its position of laxity, apply compression or traction along the femur to facilitate laxity, and follow any tissue release until completed;

Hip myofascial release

3. Direct: Move the hip into its restriction and apply gentle force until tissue give is completed;

4. Retest hip internal and external rotation; if successful and tolerated, consider prescribing HIP ABDUCTOR POSITION OF EASE or HIP ABDUCTOR STRETCH;

5. Alternative technique: Test flexion–extension, abduction–adduction, and internal–external rotation, stacking the positions of laxity or restriction and performing indirect or direct myofascial release.

HIP MYOFASCIAL RELEASE—LONG LEVER (Indirect)

INDICATIONS: Hip tension or restriction related to hip pain, low back pain, pelvic pain, gait abnormality, and other problems.

RELATIVE CONTRAINDICATIONS: Acute hip fracture or dislocation or deep venous thrombosis.

TECHNIQUE (supine):

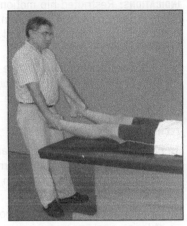
Hip myofascial release, long lever

1. Stand at the foot of the table and hold the ankles with your arms relaxed;

2. Slowly move both legs from one side to another, identifying their positions of laxity;

3. Lean backward to apply gentle traction to the legs;

4. Maintain leg positions of laxity and traction, following any tissue release until completed;

5. Retest for tension or restriction; if successful and tolerated, consider prescribing HIP ABDUCTOR POSITION OF EASE or HIP ABDUCTOR STRETCH.

HIP ABDUCTOR POSITION OF EASE

1. Lie on your back with two or three pillows placed next to the painful hip;

2. Bend the knee of the involved leg and allow it to rest on the pillows;

3. If comfortable, take a few deep breaths and rest in this position for 2–5 minutes;

4. Slowly straighten the leg;

5. Repeat 2–4 times a day, or as needed for pain relief.

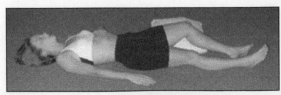
Hip abductor position of ease

HIP/PELVIS PERCUSSION VIBRATOR

INDICATIONS: Restricted hip or pelvis motion associated with hip pain, pelvic pain, back pain, gait abnormality, and other problems.

RELATIVE CONTRAINDICATIONS: Acute hip fracture or sprain, hip joint inflammation, deep venous thrombosis, lower extremity or pelvic cancer, hip replacement, or pregnancy.

TECHNIQUE (supine):

1. Place your right hand over the left greater trochanter;
2. Place the vibrating percussion pad lightly on the left greater trochanter, avoiding pad bouncing;
3. Alter pad speed, pressure, and angle until vibrations are palpated as strong by the monitoring hand;
4. Maintain contact until the force and rhythm of vibrations return to that of normal tissue;
5. Alternative technique:
   a) Allow the monitoring hand to be pulled toward the pad, resisting any other direction of hand pull;
   b) Maintain percussion until the monitoring hand is pushed away from the pad;
6. Slowly release the monitoring hand and the percussion vibrator and retest motion.

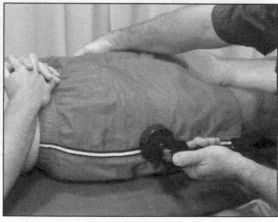

Hip percussion vibrator

HIP MUSCLE ENERGY

INDICATIONS: Restricted hip motion related to hip pain, low back pain, pelvic pain, gait abnormality, and other problems.

RELATIVE CONTRAINDICATIONS: Acute hip fracture or dislocation, acute hip sprain, hip joint inflammation, or femoral head avascular necrosis.

TECHNIQUE (supine):

1. Test hip flexion–extension, abduction–adduction, and internal–external rotation to identify restrictions;

2. Move the hip to its restrictive barrier and ask the patient to gently push the leg away from the restriction against your equal resistance for 3–5 seconds;

3. Allow full relaxation and then slowly move the hip to a new restrictive barrier;

4. Repeat this isometric contraction and stretch 3–5 times, or until motion returns;

5. Retest hip motion; if successful and tolerated, consider prescribing HAMSTRING or HIP ABDUCTOR STRETCH.

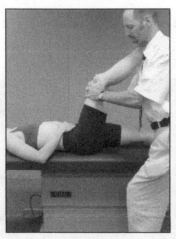

Flexion

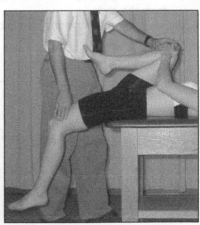

Extension

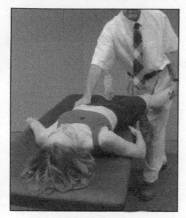

Abduction

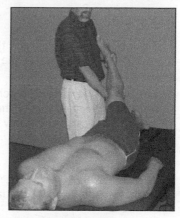

Adduction

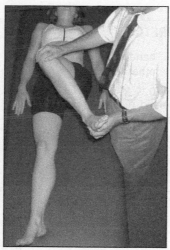

Internal rotation (external rotation opposite)

HAMSTRING STRETCH

1. Sit with one leg straight and the hand on the same side on the floor behind you;
2. Keeping the leg straight, reach with the other hand toward the foot as far as you can comfortably go;
3. Take a few deep breaths and stretch for 10–20 seconds;
4. Repeat for the other leg;
5. Do this stretch 2–4 times a day.

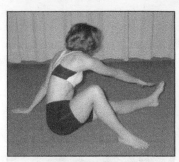

Hamstring stretch

HIP ABDUCTOR STRETCH

1. Lying on your back, bend one leg up and let it fall across the other leg;
2. Use the opposite arm to grasp the bent leg above the knee and pull it across the other leg as far as it will comfortably go;
3. Take a few deep breaths and stretch for 10–20 seconds;
4. Repeat to the other side;
5. Do this stretch 1–4 times a day.

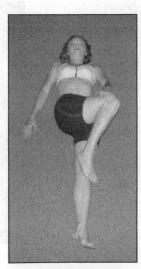

Hip abductor stretch

KNEE MOTION TESTING (active or passive)

1. With the patient seated with legs hanging, observe or test flexion and extension, comparing right and left sides;
2. Restricted flexion = extension ease = posterior tibia;
3. Restricted extension = flexion ease = anterior tibia.

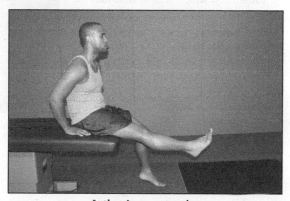

Active knee extension

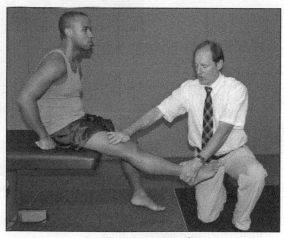

Passive knee extension

TIBIAL TORSION PALPATION

1. With the patient supine, place your thumb and index finger of one hand on the lateral margins of the patella;

2. Place the tip of your other index finger on the midline of the tibial tuberosity, which should normally be below the middle of the patella;

3. Tibial tuberosity lateral = tibia external rotation;
   Tibial tuberosity medial = tibia internal rotation.

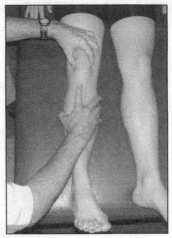

Normal tibial alignment

DRAWER TEST

1. With the patient supine, flex one knee to 90° and gently sit on the foot;

2. Grasp the proximal tibia with thumbs at tibial tuberosity and fingers posteriorly;

3. Gently pull the tibia anteriorly, comparing with the other knee if needed:

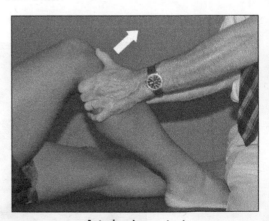

Anterior drawer test

   a) Laxity suggests anterior cruciate ligament sprain
   b) Restriction = posterior tibia

4. Gently push the tibia posteriorly, comparing with the other knee if needed:

   a) Laxity suggests posterior cruciate ligament sprain
   b) Restriction = anterior tibia.

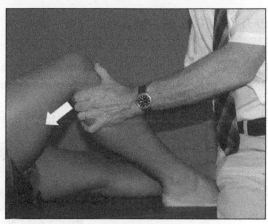

Posterior drawer test

PATELLA TENDON COUNTERSTRAIN

INDICATIONS: Patella tendon tender point associated with knee pain, leg pain, gait abnormality, and other problems.

RELATIVE CONTRAINDICATIONS: Acute knee sprain with internal derangement, acute patella fracture, or deep venous thrombosis.

TECHNIQUE (supine):

1. Place a pillow or your knee under the foot and locate the tender point in the patella tendon, labeling it 10/10;

2. Push the distal femur posterior to extend the knee and retest for tenderness;

3. Fine-tune this position with slight tibia internal or external rotation until tenderness is minimized to 0/10 if possible, but at most to 3/10;

4. Hold this position for 90 seconds, maintaining finger contact to monitor for tissue texture changes, but reducing pressure;

5. Slowly and passively return the leg to neutral and retest for tenderness using the same pressure as initial labeling. If successful, consider prescribing PATELLA POSITION OF EASE.

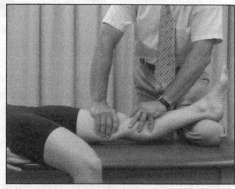

Patella tendon counterstrain

PATELLA POSITION OF EASE

1. Lie on your back with the legs straight;
2. Place a pillow or two under your foot on the side of thigh or knee pain;
3. If comfortable, take a few deep breaths and rest in this position for 2–5 minutes;
4. Use this position as often as needed for pain relief.

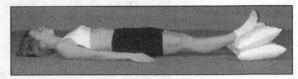

Patella position of ease

MENISCUS COUNTERSTRAIN

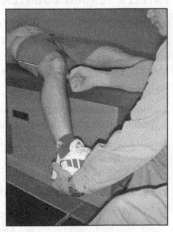

INDICATIONS: Medial or lateral meniscus tender point associated with knee pain, leg pain, gait abnormality, and other problems.

RELATIVE CONTRAINDICATIONS: Acute knee sprain with internal derangement, or deep venous thrombosis.

TECHNIQUE (supine):

1. Locate the tender point at the medial knee joint line (lateral joint line for lateral meniscus), labeling it 10/10;

Medial meniscus counterstrain

2. Hold the ankle, flex the knee about 60° by dropping the leg off the table, and retest for tenderness;
3. Fine-tune this position with slight tibia internal rotation and adduction (external rotation and abduction for lateral meniscus) until tenderness is minimized to 0/10 if possible, but at most to 3/10;
4. Hold this position for 90 seconds, maintaining finger contact to monitor for tissue texture changes, but reducing pressure;
5. Slowly and passively return the leg to neutral and retest for tenderness using the same pressure as initial labeling. If successful, consider prescribing MEDIAL MENISCUS POSITION OF EASE.

MEDIAL MENISCUS POSITION OF EASE

1. Lie on the side of the painful knee;
2. Extend the painful knee backward and rest the end of your foot on a pillow;
3. If comfortable, take a few deep breaths and rest in this position for 2–5 minutes;
4. Use this position as often as needed for pain relief.

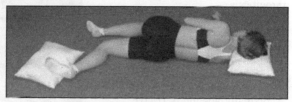

Medial meniscus position of ease

ANTERIOR CRUCIATE COUNTERSTRAIN

INDICATIONS: Anterior cruciate tender point associated with knee pain, thigh pain, gait abnormality, and other problems.

RELATIVE CONTRAINDICATIONS: Acute knee sprain with internal derangement, or deep venous thrombosis.

TECHNIQUE (supine):

1. Place a pillow under the distal femur above the knee and locate the tender point in the distal medial hamstring, labeling it 10/10;

2. Push the proximal tibia posteriorly and retest for tenderness;

3. Fine-tune with more posterior pressure and slight internal or external rotation until tenderness is minimized to 0/10 if possible, but at most to 3/10;

4. Hold this position for 90 seconds, maintaining finger contact to monitor for tissue texture changes, but reducing pressure;

5. Slowly and passively return the leg to neutral and retest for tenderness using the same pressure as initial labeling.

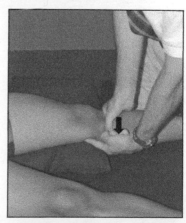

Anterior cruciate counterstrain

POSTERIOR CRUCIATE COUNTERSTRAIN

INDICATIONS: Posterior cruciate tender point associated with knee pain, thigh pain, gait abnormality, and other problems.

RELATIVE CONTRAINDICATIONS: Acute knee sprain with internal derangement, or deep venous thrombosis.

TECHNIQUE (supine):

1. Place a pillow under the proximal tibia below the knee and locate the tender point in the popliteus muscle near the posterior tibial plateau, labeling it 10/10;

2. Push the distal femur posteriorly and retest for tenderness;

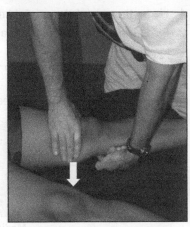

Posterior cruciate counterstrain

3. Fine-tune with more posterior pressure and slight internal or external rotation until tenderness is minimized to 0/10 if possible, but at most to 3/10;

4. Hold this position for 90 seconds, maintaining finger contact to monitor for tissue texture changes, but reducing pressure;

5. Slowly and passively return the leg to neutral and retest for tenderness using the same pressure as initial labeling.

KNEE MYOFASCIAL RELEASE

INDICATIONS: Restricted knee flexion or extension related to knee pain, leg pain, gait abnormality, and other problems.

RELATIVE CONTRAINDICATIONS: Acute fracture or deep venous thrombosis.

TECHNIQUE (supine or seated):

1. Grasp the proximal leg with your thumbs on the tibial plateau and hold the foot between your knees;

2. Move the tibia into anterior–posterior glide, medial–lateral glide, and internal–external rotation to determine directions of laxity and restriction;

3. Indirect: Slowly move the tibia to its positions of laxity and follow any tissue release until completed;

4. Direct: Slowly move the tibia into its restrictions and maintain constant force until tissue give is completed;

5. Retest tibial or knee motion; if successful and tolerated, consider prescribing HAMSTRING POSITION OF EASE or HAMSTRING STRETCH.

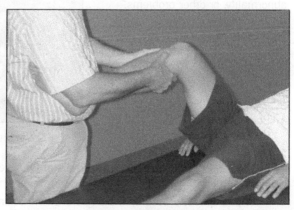

Knee myofascial release

HAMSTRING POSITION OF EASE

1. Lay face down and place a pillow or two under the ankle of the involved leg;
2. If comfortable, take a few deep breaths and rest in this position for 2–5 minutes;
3. Use this position as often as needed for pain relief.

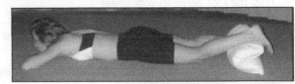

Hamstring position of ease

KNEE PERCUSSION VIBRATOR

INDICATIONS: Restricted knee or fibular head motion associated with knee pain, knee restriction, gait abnormality, or other problems.

RELATIVE CONTRAINDICATIONS: Acute knee sprain, knee joint inflammation, deep venous thrombosis, lower extremity cancer, post-knee surgery, or knee replacement.

TECHNIQUE (supine, prone, seated):

1. Place your monitoring hand over the medial knee;

Knee percussion vibrator

2. Place the vibrating percussion pad lightly on the lateral knee at the distal femur or the fibular head, avoiding pad bouncing;
3. Alter pad speed, pressure, and angle until vibrations are palpated as strong by the monitoring hand;
4. Maintain contact until the force and rhythm of vibrations returns to that of normal tissue;
5. Alternative technique:
   a) Allow the monitoring hand to be pulled toward the pad, resisting any other direction of hand pull;
   b) Maintain percussion until the monitoring hand is pushed away from the pad;
6. Slowly release the monitoring hand and the percussion vibrator and retest motion.

KNEE ARTICULATORY

INDICATIONS: Restricted tibia internal or external rotation related to knee pain, gait abnormality, and other problems.

RELATIVE CONTRAINDICATIONS: Joint inflammation, acute sprain, acute fracture, joint hypermobility, deep venous thrombosis, lower extremity cancer, or severe knee osteoarthritis.

TECHNIQUE (supine):

1. Lift the distal femur with one hand to slightly flex the knee;
2. Hold the anterior tibia below the tibial tuberosity with your other hand;
3. In one smooth motion, slowly flex the knee, rotate the tibia into its restriction, and extend the knee;
4. Repeat 3–5 times, or until joint mobility returns;
5. Retest tibial rotation; if successful and tolerated, consider prescribing PATELLA SELF-MOBILIZATION.

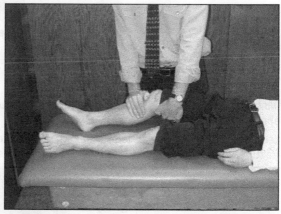

Articulatory for restricted knee internal rotation

PATELLA SELF-MOBILIZATION[2]

1. Sit with your legs straight and a hand on the floor behind you;
2. Use the web of your other hand to push the involved kneecap down toward the big toe as far as it will comfortably go;
3. Gently push the lower leg up toward the ceiling until knee pain occurs;
4. Release and repeat 2–5 times;
5. Perform this mobilization 2–4 times a day.

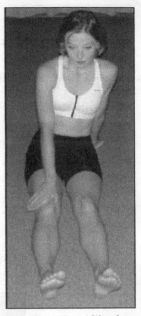

Patella self-mobilization

ANTERIOR TIBIA THRUST

INDICATIONS: Restricted knee extension related to knee pain, gait abnormality, or other problems.

RELATIVE CONTRAINDICATIONS: Joint inflammation, acute sprain, acute fracture, joint hypermobility, deep venous thrombosis, lower extremity cancer, or severe knee osteoarthritis.

TECHNIQUE (supine):

1. Flex the knee to 90° and gently sit on the foot;
2. Grasp the proximal tibia with thumbs at tibial tuberosity and fingers posteriorly;
3. Gently push the tibia to the posterior glide restrictive barrier;
4. Ask the patient to take a deep breath and during exhalation apply a short and quick posterior thrust along the knee joint line;
5. Retest tibia motion.

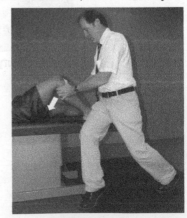

Anterior tibia thrust

POSTERIOR TIBIA THRUST

INDICATIONS: Restricted knee flexion related to knee pain, gait abnormality, and other problems.

RELATIVE CONTRAINDICATIONS: Joint inflammation, acute sprain, acute fracture, joint hypermobility, deep venous thrombosis, lower extremity cancer, or severe knee osteoarthritis.

TECHNIQUE (prone):

1. Flex the knee to 90° and place the foot on your shoulder;

2. Grasp the proximal tibia with fingers intertwined behind the knee;

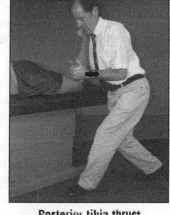
Posterior tibia thrust

3. Gently pull the tibia to the anterior glide restrictive barrier;

4. Ask the patient to take a deep breath and during exhalation apply a short and quick inferior thrust;

5. Retest tibia motion.

ANKLE MOTION

1. With the patient supine or seated, induce dorsiflexion and plantar flexion, comparing the range for right and left ankles;

2. Restricted dorsiflexion = anterior talus;
   Restricted plantar flexion = posterior talus.

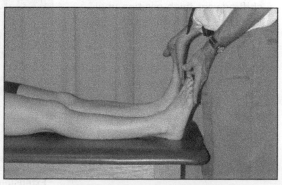
Left ankle restricted dorsiflexion

ANKLE SWING TEST

1. With the patient seated, grasp the feet with your thumbs on the anterior talus;

2. Push the feet posteriorly while holding them horizontal to glide the talus posteriorly and dorsiflex the ankles, comparing sides for restricted motion;

3. Positive swing test = restricted posterior talus glide = anterior talus = plantar flexion somatic dysfunction.

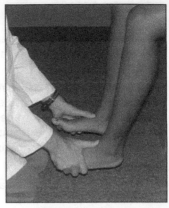

Ankle swing test

EXTENSION ANKLE COUNTERSTRAIN

INDICATIONS: Tender point in gastrocnemius muscle associated with ankle pain, leg pain, foot pain, gait abnormality, and other problems.

RELATIVE CONTRAINDICATIONS: Acute ankle sprain with joint instability, acute fracture, or deep venous thrombosis.

TECHNIQUE (prone):

1. Locate the tender point in the proximal gastrocnemius muscle near its medial or lateral origin, labeling it 10/10;

2. Flex the patient's knee, place your foot on the table, rest the patient's foot on your thigh, and retest for tenderness;

3. Fine-tune this position by pushing the patient's foot into your thigh and shifting your thigh position until tenderness is minimized to 0/10 if possible, but at most to 3/10;

4. Hold this position for 90 seconds, maintaining finger contact to monitor for tissue texture changes, but reducing pressure;

5. Slowly and passively return the leg to neutral and retest for tenderness using the same pressure as initial labeling. If successful, consider prescribing ACHILLES/GASTROCNEMIUS POSITION OF EASE.

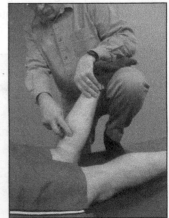

Extension ankle counterstrain

ACHILLES/GASTROCNEMIUS POSITION OF EASE

1. Lay face down with the involved foot resting on a pillow or two;
2. If comfortable, take a few deep breaths and rest in this position for 2–5 minutes;
3. Repeat 2–4 times a day, or as needed for pain relief.

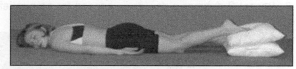

Achilles/gastrocnemius position of ease

LATERAL ANKLE COUNTERSTRAIN

INDICATIONS: Lateral ankle tender point associated with ankle pain, leg pain, foot pain, gait abnormality, and other problems.

RELATIVE CONTRAINDICATIONS: Acute ankle sprain with joint instability, acute fracture, or deep venous thrombosis.

TECHNIQUE (lateral):

1. With the patient lying on the side of the problem, use one hand to hold the distal tibia and locate the tender point anterior and inferior to the lateral malleolus, labeling it 10/10;
2. Hold the calcaneus with your other hand, evert the foot by pushing the calcaneus toward the floor, and retest for tenderness;
3. Fine-tune this position with slightly more or less eversion until tenderness is minimized to 0/10 if possible, but at most to 3/10;
4. Hold this position for 90 seconds, maintaining finger contact to monitor for tissue texture changes, but reducing pressure;
5. Slowly and passively return the foot to neutral and retest for tenderness using the same pressure as initial labeling. If successful, consider prescribing LATERAL ANKLE POSITION OF EASE.

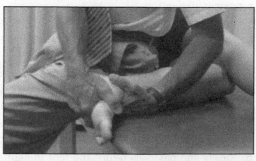

Lateral ankle counterstrain

LATERAL ANKLE POSITION OF EASE

1. Lie on the side of ankle pain with a pillow under your leg and the foot hanging off the end of the pillow;
2. If comfortable, take a few deep breaths and rest in this position for 2–5 minutes;
3. Repeat 2–4 times a day, or as needed for pain relief.

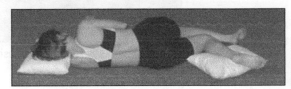

Lateral ankle position of ease

MEDIAL ANKLE COUNTERSTRAIN

INDICATIONS: Medial ankle tender point associated with ankle pain, leg pain, foot pain, gait abnormality, and other problems.

RELATIVE CONTRAINDI-CATIONS: Acute ankle sprain with joint instability, acute fracture, or deep venous thrombosis.

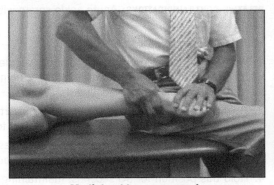

Medial ankle counterstrain

TECHNIQUE (lateral):

1. With the patient lying on the opposite side of the problem, use one hand to hold the distal tibia and locate the tender point inferior to the medial malleolus, labeling it 10/10;
2. Invert the foot with your other hand and retest for tenderness;
3. Fine-tune this position with slight foot internal rotation and inversion until tenderness minimized to 0/10 if possible, but at most to 3/10;
4. Hold this position for 90 seconds, maintaining finger contact to monitor for tissue texture changes, but reducing pressure;
5. Slowly and passively return the foot to neutral and retest for tenderness using the same pressure as initial labeling.

ANKLE MYOFASCIAL RELEASE

INDICATIONS: Restricted ankle motion related to ankle pain, leg pain, foot pain, gait abnormality, and other problems.

RELATIVE CONTRAINDICATIONS: Acute fracture or dislocation, calf deep venous thrombosis, or acute sprain (direct).

TECHNIQUE (seated or supine):

1. Hold the calcaneus and plantar surface of the foot with one hand and distal leg with the other;
2. Test ankle dorsiflexion and plantar flexion, comparing with the other side to determine directions of laxity and restriction;
3. Indirect: Gently and slowly move the ankle to its position of laxity, apply compression or traction between your hands to facilitate laxity, and follow any tissue release until it is completed;
4. Direct (contraindicated for acute sprain): Slowly move the ankle into its restriction and apply steady force until tissue give is completed;
5. Slowly return the ankle to neutral and retest motion.

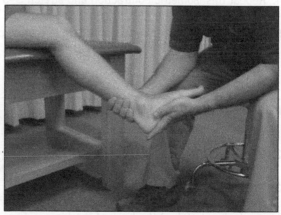

Ankle myofascial release

ANKLE MUSCLE ENERGY

INDICATIONS: Restricted ankle motion related to ankle pain, leg pain, foot pain, gait abnormality, and other problems.

RELATIVE CONTRAINDICATIONS: Acute fracture or dislocation, acute sprain, ankle joint inflammation, or calf deep venous thrombosis.

TECHNIQUE (seated or supine):

1. Test ankle dorsiflexion and plantar flexion, comparing both sides to identify a restriction;

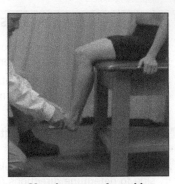

Muscle energy for ankle dorsiflexion restriction

2. Move the ankle to its restrictive barrier, and ask the patient to gently push or pull the foot away from the restriction against your equal resistance for 3–5 seconds;

3. Allow full relaxation and then slowly move the ankle to a new restrictive barrier;

4. Repeat this isometric contraction and stretch 3–5 times, or until motion returns;

5. Retest ankle motion; if successful and tolerated, consider prescribing ACHILLES/GASTROCNEMIUS STRETCH.

ACHILLES/GASTROCNEMIUS STRETCH

1. Stand 3–4 feet from a wall;

2. Step toward the wall with one leg, placing your hands on the wall;

3. Keep the heel of your back leg on the floor and slowly lean into the wall until you feel a stretch at the back of the leg;

4. Take a few deep breaths and stretch for 10–20 seconds;

5. Repeat this stretch with the involved knee slightly bent;

6. Repeat for the other leg;

7. Do these stretches 2–4 times a day.

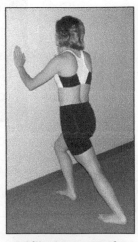

Achilles/gastrocnemius stretch

ANKLE THRUST

INDICATIONS: Restricted ankle dorsiflexion related to ankle pain, leg pain, foot pain, gait abnormality, and other problems.

RELATIVE CONTRAINDICATIONS: Acute fracture or dislocation, acute sprain, ankle joint inflammation, ankle joint hypermobility, or calf deep venous thrombosis.

TECHNIQUE (supine):

1. Stand at the foot of the table and grasp the foot with your fifth fingers on the dorsal talus and thumbs on the plantar surface near the distal metatarsal heads;

2. Evert the foot and move the ankle to its dorsiflexion restrictive barrier;

3. Ask the patient to take a deep breath and, during exhalation, apply a short and quick caudad tug of the foot while maintaining the dorsiflexion barrier;

4. Retest ankle dorsiflexion.

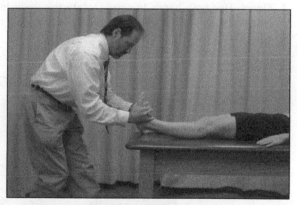

Thrust for ankle dorsiflexion restriction

INTEROSSEOUS MEMBRANE MYOFASCIAL RELEASE

INDICATIONS: Restricted leg fascial rotation related to leg pain, ankle pain, gait abnormality, and other problems. The technique can be adapted for restricted forearm fascia rotation related to arm pain and other problems.

RELATIVE CONTRAINDICATIONS: Acute sprain, acute fracture, or deep venous thrombosis.

TECHNIQUE (supine):

1. Hold the proximal leg at the tibial tuberosity and fibular head with one hand and the distal leg at the lateral and medial malleoli with the other;
2. Rotate the hands in opposite directions and then reverse directions to determine torsional laxity versus restriction;
3. Indirect: Use both hands to slowly rotate the lower leg into its position of torsional laxity, apply compression or traction between your hands to facilitate laxity, and follow any tissue release until completed;
4. Direct: Use both hands to slowly rotate the lower leg into its torsional restriction and apply steady force until tissue give is completed;
5. Retest rotational torsion.

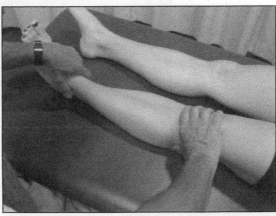

Interosseous membrane myofascial release

FIBULAR HEAD MOTION

1. With the patient supine and knees bent, place your thumb and index finger on the anterior and posterior sides of the proximal fibular head;

2. Pull the fibular head anterolaterally and push it posteromedially to identify joint glide;

3. Restricted anterolateral glide = posterior fibular head; Restricted posteromedial glide = anterior fibular head.

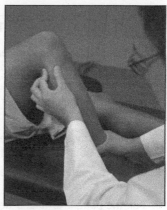

Fibular head motion

FIBULAR HEAD MUSCLE ENERGY

INDICATIONS: Fibular head restriction associated with knee pain, fibular neuritis (see FIBULAR NERVE, *p. 58*), ankle pain, gait abnormality, and other problems.

RELATIVE CONTRAINDICATIONS: Acute ankle sprain, acute fibular fracture, deep venous thrombosis, or ankle joint laxity.

TECHNIQUE (supine or seated):

1. Flex the knee about 90°;

2. Pull the fibular head anterolaterally while dorsiflexing the foot to its restrictive barrier;

3. Ask the patient to plantar flex the foot against your equal resistance for 3–5 seconds;

4. Allow full relaxation and slowly move the ankle to a new dorsiflexion barrier as you continue pulling the fibular head anterolaterally;

5. Repeat this isometric contraction and stretch 3–5 times, or until fibular head mobility returns;

6. Retest fibular head motion;

7. For an anterior fibular head, push the fibular head posteromedially in steps 2 and 4.

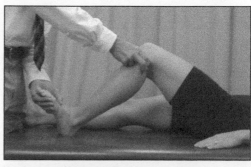

Fibular head muscle energy

ANTERIOR FIBULAR HEAD THRUST

INDICATIONS: Anterior fibular head associated with lower extremity pain, gait abnormality, and other problems.

RELATIVE CONTRAINDICATIONS: Acute fibular fracture, deep venous thrombosis, knee instability, or knee inflammation.

TECHNIQUE (supine):

1. Place your thenar eminence on the anterior fibular head and grasp the distal tibia with your other hand;
2. Push the fibular head posteromedially by leaning into it with a rigid arm as you internally rotate the tibia to engage the restrictive barrier;
3. Ask the patient to take a deep breath and, during exhalation, apply a short and quick posteromedial thrust into the fibular head;
4. Retest fibular head motion.

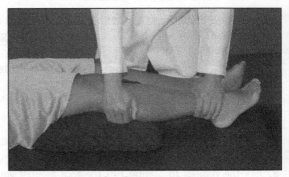

Anterior fibular head thrust

POSTERIOR FIBULAR HEAD THRUST

INDICATIONS: Posterior fibular head associated with lower extremity pain, fibular neuritis (see FIBULAR NERVE, *p. 58*), gait abnormality, and other problems.

RELATIVE CONTRAINDICATIONS: Acute ankle sprain, acute fibular fracture, deep venous thrombosis, knee instability, or knee inflammation.

TECHNIQUE (supine):

1. Place your first metacarpal–phalangeal joint posteromedial to the posterior fibular head and grasp the tibia with your other hand;

2. Externally rotate the tibia to the restrictive barrier and flex the knee until your hand is wedged between the posterior fibular head and thigh;

3. Ask the patient to take a deep breath and during exhalation apply a quick short thrust by flexing the knee;

4. Retest fibular head motion.

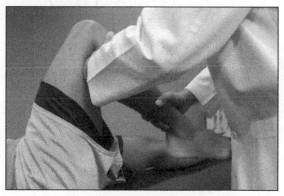

Posterior fibular head thrust

Fibular Nerve

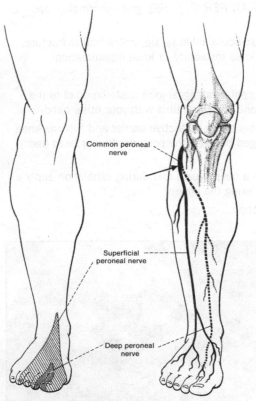

Common peroneal nerve

Superficial peroneal nerve

Deep peroneal nerve

Fibular (common peroneal) nerve is compressed by posterior fibular head

CALCANEUS COUNTERSTRAIN

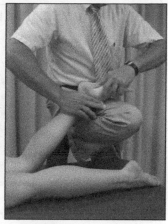

Calcaneus counterstrain

INDICATIONS: Calcaneus tender point associated with foot pain, ankle pain, gait abnormality, and other problems.

RELATIVE CONTRAINDICATIONS: Acute ankle sprain with joint instability, acute fracture, or deep venous thrombosis.

TECHNIQUE (prone):

1. Locate the tender point on the bottom of the foot at the distal edge of the calcaneus, labeling it 10/10;

2. Flex the patient's knee, place your foot on the table, rest the patient's foot on your thigh, and retest for tenderness;

3. Fine-tune this position by pushing the patient's leg into your thigh, shifting your thigh position, and slightly inverting or everting the foot until tenderness is minimized to 0/10 if possible, but at most to 3/10;

4. Hold this position for 90 seconds, maintaining finger contact to monitor for tissue texture changes, but reducing pressure;

5. Slowly and passively return the foot to neutral and retest for tenderness using the same pressure as initial labeling.

FOREFOOT MYOFASCIAL RELEASE

INDICATIONS: Restricted forefoot inversion or eversion related to foot pain, ankle pain, gait abnormality, and other problems.

RELATIVE CONTRAINDICATIONS: Acute fracture or dislocation.

TECHNIQUE (seated or supine):

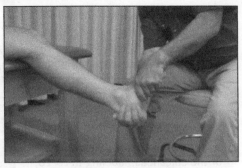

Forefoot myofascial release

1. Hold the calcaneus firmly with one hand and the forefoot with the other, at the level of the proximal tarsal–metatarsal joints;

2. Test forefoot inversion and eversion to determine directions of ease and restriction, comparing with the other foot if needed;

3. Indirect: Gently and slowly move the forefoot to its position of laxity, apply compression or traction between your hands to facilitate laxity, and follow any tissue release until it is completed;

4. Direct: Slowly move the forefoot into its restriction and apply steady force until tissue give is completed;

5. Slowly return the forefoot to neutral and retest motion.

FOOT ARTICULATORY

INDICATIONS: Metatarsal joint restriction associated with foot pain, ankle pain, gait abnormality, and other problems.

RELATIVE CONTRAINDICATIONS: Acute fracture or sprain, joint inflammation, or joint hypermobility.

TECHNIQUE (supine):

1. Stabilize the proximal bone of the joint being treated with one hand;

Articulatory for first and second tarsal–metatarsal joints

2. Grasp the distal bone with your other hand and gently test superior and inferior glide;

3. If restricted, slowly circumduct the distal bone clockwise and counterclockwise 3–5 times, or until motion returns;

4. Retest metatarsal motion.

TARSAL THRUST (Hiss Whip)

INDICATIONS: Navicular or cuboid tenderness and restriction associated with foot pain, ankle pain, gait abnormality, and other problems.

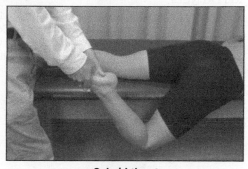

Cuboid thrust

RELATIVE CONTRAINDICATIONS: Acute fracture or sprain, joint inflammation, or joint hypermobility.

TECHNIQUE (prone or standing):

1. Hold the foot with both thumbs on the medial aspect of the navicular or cuboid bone;
2. Flex the hip and knee by dropping the leg off the table;
3. Plantar flex the ankle and push the tarsal bone to its restrictive barrier:
   Navicular—push dorsally and medially;
   Cuboid—push dorsally and laterally;
4. Apply a short and quick thrust with the thumbs into the restrictive barrier while swinging the ankle into plantar flexion;
5. Retest arch flexibility (tenderness may not be alleviated immediately).

INTERPHALANGEAL ARTICULATORY (Foot or Hand)

INDICATIONS: Interphalangeal restriction associated with foot or hand pain and other related problems.

RELATIVE CONTRAINDICATIONS: Acute fracture or sprain, joint inflammation, or joint hypermobility.

TECHNIQUE (seated or supine):

1. Stabilize the proximal bone of the joint being treated with one hand;
2. Grasp the distal bone with your other hand and gently flex and extend it to identify motion restriction;
3. Apply traction to the distal bone and slowly circumduct it in both directions 3–5 times, or until motion returns;
4. Retest interphalangeal motion.

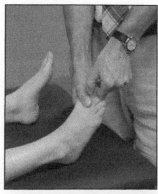

Articulatory for second PIP joint

REFERENCES

1. Glossary Review Committee (ECOP of AACOM). *Glossary of Osteopathic Terminology*. Chevy Chase, MD: Educational Council on Osteopathic Principles of the American Association of Colleges of Osteopathic Medicine; 2009.
2. Baycroft CM. A self-treatment method for patello-femoral dysfunction. *J Manual Med*. 1990;5:25–26.

4 Pelvis Diagnosis and Treatment

Diagnosis of Pelvis Somatic Dysfunction:
1. Screening tests
   Standing flexion test *p. 64*
   ASIS compression test *p. 64*
   Pelvis diagnosis using inherent motion *p. 65*
2. Pelvis palpation—anterior *p. 66*
3. Pelvis palpation—posterior *p. 67*
4. Pelvis somatic dysfunction (Table 4-1) *p. 68*

Treatment of Pelvis Somatic Dysfunction:
1. OMT
   High ilium counterstrain *p. 68*
   High ilium flare-out counterstrain *p. 69*
   Low ilium counterstrain *p. 70*
   Iliopsoas counterstrain *p. 71*
   Lumbosacral myofascial release *p. 74*
   Pelvis percussion vibrator *p. 75*
   Sacroiliac-seated facet release *p. 76*
   Anterior innominate muscle energy *p. 77*
   Anterior innominate thrust—lateral recumbent *p. 78*
   Anterior innominate thrust—supine *p. 79*
   Posterior innominate muscle energy *p. 80*
   Posterior innominate thrust—lateral recumbent *p. 82*
   Posterior innominate thrust—supine *p. 83*
   Pubic muscle energy/thrust *p. 84*
   Ilium inflare muscle energy *p. 86*
   Ilium outflare muscle energy *p. 87*
   Sacroiliac articulatory *p. 88*
2. Exercises
   Iliopsoas position of ease *p. 73*
   Iliopsoas stretch *p. 73*
   Quadriceps stretch *p. 81*
   Pubic self-mobilization *p. 85*

63

Diagnosis

SCREENING TESTS

Standing Flexion Test

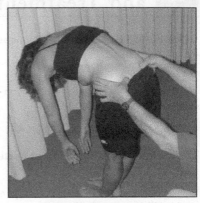

1. Place your thumbs on the undersurface of the posterior superior iliac spines (PSIS) of the standing patient, taking care to keep both thumbs horizontal;

2. Ask the patient to bend forward with the legs straight and allow your thumbs to follow PSIS movement, taking care to maintain both thumbs underneath the PSIS;

Standing flexion test

3. The side on which the PSIS stops moving superiorly the last is the side of pelvis restriction at the sacroiliac joint;

4. False positives: contralateral hamstring tightness; short leg; sacral, lumbar, 12th rib, and other somatic dysfunctions on the same side.

ASIS Compression Test

1. With the patient supine, place your palms on the anterior superior iliac spines (ASIS);

2. Push posteromedially on one ASIS at a time, comparing the resistance of the two sides;

3. Resistance to posteromedial pressure indicates sacroiliac joint restriction on that side.

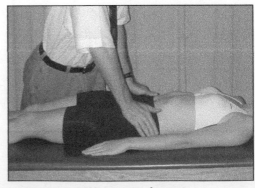

ASIS compression test

Pelvis Diagnosis Using Inherent Motion*

1. With the patient supine, place your hands gently over the ilia with palms on ASIS and fingers inferior to iliac crests;

2. Palpate inherent external and internal rotation to identify restricted motion;

   a) Restricted bilateral external rotation indicates inherent extension;
   b) Restricted unilateral external rotation indicates anterior innominate or internally rotated ilium;
   c) Restricted bilateral internal rotation indicates inherent flexion;
   d) Restricted unilateral internal rotation indicates posterior innominate or externally rotated ilium;

3. If related to the patient problem, treat the restriction with myofascial release, balanced membranous tension, or other techniques.

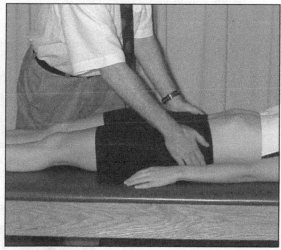

Palpation for inherent external/internal rotation

---

*The term *inherent motion* refers to a palpable cyclic pressure fluctuation variably referred to as cranial rhythmic impulse, craniosacral motion, entrainment, primary respiratory mechanism, pulse pressure fluctuation, and Traube–Hering–Mayer wave.

PELVIS PALPATION—ANTERIOR

1. Palpate for tenderness at the following locations:
   a) **Iliacus tender point**—1" medial and slightly inferior to ASIS (see ILIOPSOAS MUSCLE, *p. 72*);
   b) Pubic symphysis—anterior surface.
2. Palpate for symmetry at the following locations after seating the pelvis:
   a) Seating the pelvis—Have the supine patient bend the knees, place the feet on the table, lift the pelvis off the table and set it down, and straighten the legs;
   b) ASIS levelness—Place your thumbs on the undersurface of the ASIS and compare for superior–inferior and medial–lateral levelness, naming for the side of pelvis restriction;
   c) Pubic tubercle levelness—Place your thumbs on the superior surface of the pubic tubercles located 1/4"–1/2" lateral to the symphysis and compare for superior–inferior levelness, naming for the side of pelvis restriction.

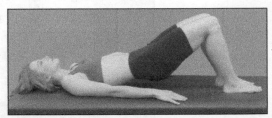

Seating the pelvis before anterior palpation

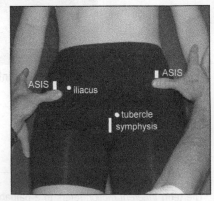

**Anterior pelvis palpation
(ASIS asymmetry shown)**

PELVIS PALPATION—POSTERIOR

1. Palpate for tender points at the following locations:
   a) **Piriformis**—musculature halfway between greater trochanter and the middle of the sacral border.
2. Palpate for symmetry at the following locations after seating the pelvis:
   a) Seating the pelvis—With the patient prone, lift the legs to flex the knees as far as they will comfortably go and then return the legs to the table;
   b) PSIS levelness—Place your thumbs on the undersurface of the PSIS and compare for superior–inferior and medial–lateral levelness, naming for the side of pelvis restriction.

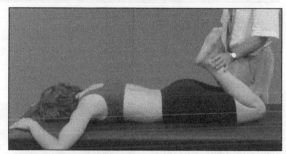

Seating the pelvis before posterior palpation

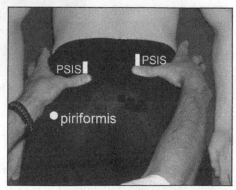

Posterior pelvis palpation
(PSIS asymmetry shown)

Table 4-1 | PELVIS SOMATIC DYSFUNCTION

Positional Diagnosis	ASIS	PSIS	Pubic Symphysis	Pubic Tubercle
Anterior innominate	Inferior	Superior	–	–
Posterior innominate	Superior	Inferior	–	–
Ilium inflare	Medial	–	–	–
Ilium outflare	Lateral	–	–	–
Superior innominate shear	Superior	Superior	–	–
Inferior innominate shear	Inferior	Inferior	–	–
Pubic compression	–	–	Tender	Symmetrical
Superior pubic shear	–	–	Tender	Superior
Inferior pubic shear			Tender	Inferior

Treatment

HIGH ILIUM COUNTERSTRAIN

INDICATIONS: High ilium tender point associated with back pain, pelvis pain, hip pain, and other problems.

RELATIVE CONTRAINDICATIONS: Acute hip fracture, hip dislocation, or severe hip osteoarthritis.

TECHNIQUE (prone):

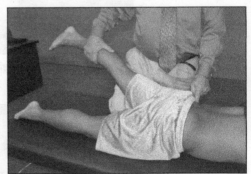

Counterstrain for left high ilium tender point

1. Locate the tender point 1" lateral to the posterior superior iliac spine, labeling it 10/10;

2. Stand on the side of the tender point and extend the hip by placing your knee under the patient's thigh;

3. Retest for tenderness and fine-tune with slight abduction or adduction until tenderness is minimized to 0/10 if possible, but at most to 3/10;

4. Hold this position of maximum relief for 90 seconds, maintaining finger contact, to monitor for tissue texture changes but reducing pressure;

5. Slowly and passively lower the leg to the table and retest for tenderness with the same pressure as initial labeling.

HIGH ILIUM FLARE-OUT COUNTERSTRAIN

INDICATIONS: High ilium flare-out tender point associated with back pain, pelvis pain, hip pain, and other problems.

RELATIVE CONTRAINDICATIONS: Acute hip fracture, hip dislocation, or severe hip osteoarthritis.

TECHNIQUE (prone):

1. Locate the tender point on the inferior lateral angle of the sacrum, labeling it 10/10;

2. Stand on the opposite side and lift the thigh on the side of the tender point to extend the hip;

3. Retest for tenderness and fine-tune with hip adduction until tenderness is 0/10 if possible, but at most to 3/10;

4. Hold this position of maximum relief for 90 seconds, maintaining finger contact to monitor for tissue texture changes, but reducing pressure;

5. Slowly and passively lower the leg to the table and retest for tenderness with the same pressure as initial labeling.

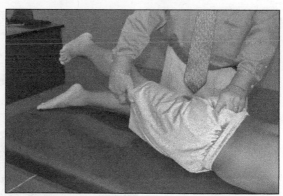

Counterstrain for right high ilium flare-out

LOW ILIUM COUNTERSTRAIN

INDICATIONS: Low ilium tender point associated with abdominal pain, pelvis pain, hip pain, back pain, and other problems.

RELATIVE CONTRAINDICATIONS: Acute lumbar or hip fracture, or hip dislocation.

TECHNIQUE (supine):

1. Stand beside the patient and locate the tender point pushing inferiorly onto the superior surface of the lateral pubic ramus, labeling it 10/10;

2. Flex the knee and hip as far as comfortable on the side of the tender point;

3. Retest for tenderness and fine-tune in all planes of motion until tenderness is 0/10 if possible, but at most to 3/10;

4. Hold this position of maximum relief for 90 seconds, maintaining finger contact to monitor for tissue texture changes, but reducing pressure;

5. Slowly and passively lower the legs to the table and retest for tenderness with the same pressure as initial labeling.

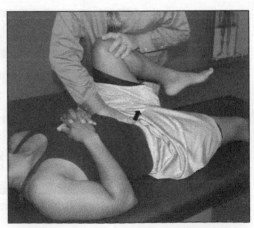

Counterstrain for left low ilium tender point

ILIOPSOAS COUNTERSTRAIN

INDICATIONS: Iliacus or psoas tender point associated with abdominal pain, pelvic pain, back pain, and other problems (see ILIOPSOAS MUSCLE, p. 72).

RELATIVE CONTRAINDICATIONS: Acute lumbar or hip fracture, or hip dislocation.

TECHNIQUE (supine):

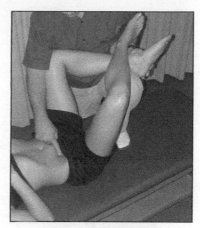

Psoas tender point and counterstrain position

1. Stand beside the patient and locate the tender point 1" medial and slightly inferior to the ASIS, labeling it 10/10;

2. Cross the ankles and passively flex the knees and hips 90°, allowing the hips to externally rotate;

3. Retest for tenderness and fine-tune this position with increased hip flexion until tenderness is 0/10 if possible, but at most to 3/10;

4. Hold the position of maximum relief for 90 seconds, maintaining finger contact to monitor for tissue texture changes but reducing pressure;

5. Slowly and passively return the legs to the table and retest for tenderness with the same pressure as initial labeling; if successful, consider prescribing ILIOPSOAS POSITION OF EASE and/or ILIOPSOAS STRETCH.

ILIOPSOAS MUSCLE

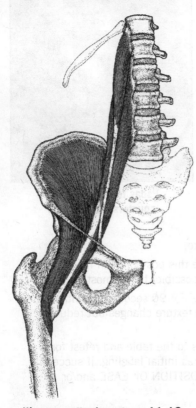

Iliopsoas attachments on L1, L2, ilium, and lesser trochanter

ILIOPSOAS POSITION OF EASE

1. Lie on your back with legs propped up on a chair or stool;
2. Cross your ankles with the foot on the side of the back or pelvic pain on top;
3. Let your knees fall apart;
4. If comfortable, take a few deep breaths and rest in this position for 2–5 minutes;
5. Slowly uncross your legs, bring them down, and roll to one side before getting up;

   Use this position 2–4 times a day, or as needed for pain relief.

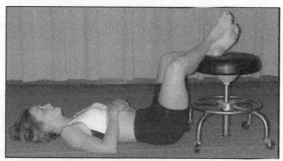

Iliopsoas position of ease

ILIOPSOAS STRETCH[1]

1. Kneel with one foot on the floor a few feet in front of the other knee;
2. Slowly lean forward onto the leg in front while using your hand to push the other hip forward;
3. Take a few deep breaths and stretch for 10–20 seconds;
4. Repeat to the opposite side;
5. Do this stretch 1–4 times a day.

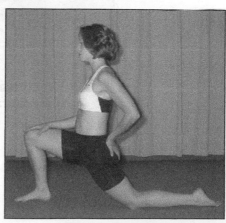

Left iliopsoas stretch

LUMBOSACRAL MYOFASCIAL RELEASE (PELVIC DIAPHRAGM)

INDICATIONS: Restricted lumbosacral fascia rotation related to low back pain, pelvic pain, edema, and other problems.

RELATIVE CONTRAINDICATIONS: Acute pelvic fracture.

TECHNIQUE (supine or prone):

1. Place your palms over the lateral pelvis and simultaneously lift one side while pushing the other side posteriorly to induce lumbosacral fascia rotation;

2. Repeat for the other direction to identify rotational restriction and laxity;

3. Indirect: Rotate the lumbosacral fascia to its position of laxity and follow any tissue release until completed;

4. Direct: Rotate the lumbosacral fascia into its restriction and apply steady force until tissue give is completed;

5. Retest lumbosacral fascia rotation.

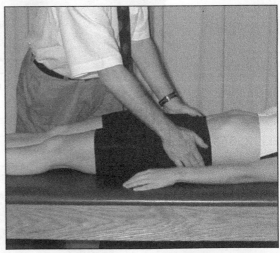

Lumbosacral myofascial release

PELVIS PERCUSSION VIBRATOR

INDICATIONS: Restricted pelvis motion associated with hip pain, pelvic pain, back pain, and other problems.

RELATIVE CONTRAINDICATIONS: Acute pelvis fracture, sacroiliitis, deep venous thrombosis, intrapelvic cancer, recent pelvic surgery, or pregnancy.

TECHNIQUE (lateral):

1. With the patient lying on the nonrestricted side with knees and hips flexed, place your monitoring hand over the iliac crest;

2. Place the vibrating percussion pad lightly on the ischial tuberosity, avoiding pad bouncing;

3. Alter pad speed, pressure, and angle until vibrations are palpated as strong by the monitoring hand;

4. Maintain contact until the force and rhythm of vibration returns to that of normal tissue.

5. Alternative technique:

   a) Allow the monitoring hand to be pulled toward the pad, resisting any other direction of hand pull;

   b) Maintain percussion until the monitoring hand is pushed away from the pad;

6. Slowly release the monitoring hand and the percussion vibrator and retest motion.

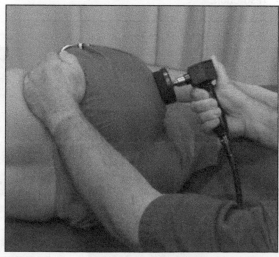

Pelvis percussion vibrator

SACROILIAC SEATED FACET RELEASE

INDICATIONS: Restricted sacroiliac joint (SIJ) motion associated with back pain, pelvic pain, and other problems.

RELATIVE CONTRAINDICATIONS: Acute pelvis fracture.

TECHNIQUE:

1. Sit behind the patient and have him or her markedly increase lumbar lordosis so that the shoulders are balanced over the pelvis;

2. Place the thumb on the inferior PSIS of the restricted sacroiliac joint;

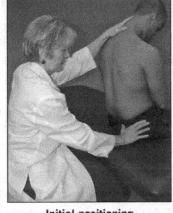

Initial positioning

3. Place your other hand on the shoulder and gently compress inferiorly while extending the lumbar spine, keeping the shoulders balanced over the pelvis;

4. Test for the position of greatest restriction by gentle compression and recoil on the shoulder to close or open the locked sacroiliac joint;

5. Hold the patient in the position of greatest restriction and gently induce a small degree of additional compression or traction through the shoulder to induce glide of the facet, thereby releasing the restriction;

6. Retest sacroiliac motion.

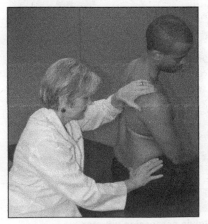

Compression for right SIJ

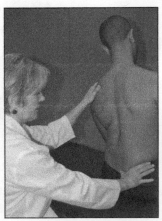

Traction for right SIJ

ANTERIOR INNOMINATE MUSCLE ENERGY

INDICATIONS: Anterior innominate rotation or inferior pubic shear associated with back pain, pelvic pain, hip pain, short leg syndrome, and other problems.

RELATIVE CONTRAINDICATIONS: Acute pelvis fracture, sacroiliac joint inflammation, or severe hip arthritis.

TECHNIQUE (supine):

1. Stand beside the involved side, flex and adduct the hip to its restrictive barrier, and pull the ischial tuberosity anteriorly. For inferior pubic shear push the ischial tuberosity superiorly;

2. Ask the patient to push the knee into your shoulder for 3–5 seconds against your equal resistance;

3. Allow full relaxation and then slowly pull the ischial tuberosity anteriorly and flex the hip to new restrictive barriers;

4. Repeat this isometric contraction and stretch 3–5 times, or until pelvic mobility returns.

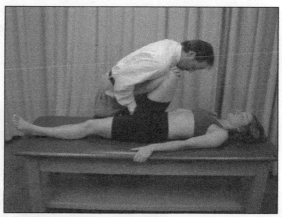

Muscle energy for right anterior innominate

ANTERIOR INNOMINATE THRUST—LATERAL RECUMBENT

INDICATIONS: Anterior innominate rotation associated with back pain, hip pain, short leg syndrome, and other problems.

RELATIVE CONTRAINDICATIONS: Acute lumbar sprain, undiagnosed radiculopathy, acute vertebral fracture, acute herniated or ruptured disc, spondylosis, sacroiliitis, or sacroiliac joint hypermobility.

TECHNIQUE:

1. Stand in front of the patient who is lying with the involved pelvis upward;
2. Flex the involved hip to 90° and drop the leg off the table;
3. Rotate the back toward the table by lifting the table-side arm until you feel rotation at the lumbosacral junction;
4. Use your cephalad arm to stabilize the shoulder, place your other forearm across the ischial tuberosity, and lean over top of that arm;
5. Ask the patient to take a deep breath and during exhalation slowly push the ischial tuberosity toward the femur to take up the rotational slack;
6. At the end of exhalation apply a short quick thrust with your arm and body onto the ischial tuberosity and toward the femur;
7. Recheck sacroiliac mobility or pelvis symmetry; if successful, consider prescribing SACROILIAC SELF-MOBILIZATION on p. 110 (in Chapter 5).

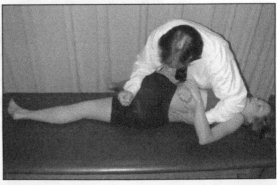

Lateral recumbent thrust for left anterior innominate

ANTERIOR INNOMINATE THRUST—SUPINE

INDICATIONS: Anterior innominate rotation associated with back pain, pelvis pain, hip pain, short leg syndrome, and other problems.

RELATIVE CONTRAINDICATIONS: Acute sacroiliac sprain, hip or knee instability, or sacroiliac joint hypermobility.

TECHNIQUE:

1. Stand at the foot of the table and grasp the leg just above the ankle with both hands above the malleoli;

2. Lift the leg to about 30° hip flexion and slightly abduct and internally rotate the leg;

3. Ask the patient to take a deep breath, and during exhalation, apply a firm and quick caudad tug down the leg;

4. Retest sacroiliac motion or pelvis symmetry; if successful, consider prescribing SACROILIAC SELF-MOBILIZATION on p. 110 (in Chapter 5).

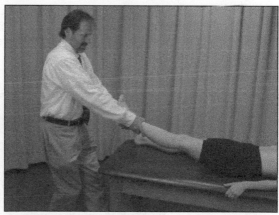

Traction tug for left anterior innominate rotation

POSTERIOR INNOMINATE MUSCLE ENERGY

INDICATIONS: Posterior innominate rotation or superior pubic shear associated with back pain, pelvic pain, hip pain, short leg syndrome, and other problems.

RELATIVE CONTRAINDICATIONS: Acute pelvic fracture, sacroiliac joint inflammation, or severe hip arthritis.

TECHNIQUE (supine):

1. Stand on the involved side and hold the opposite anterior superior iliac spine;

2. Move the involved leg off the table and allow the leg to drop to the hip extension restrictive barrier. For superior pubic shear the ischial tuberosity should remain on the table;

3. Ask the patient to push the thigh upward for 3–5 seconds against your equal resistance;

4. Allow full relaxation and then slowly extend the hip to a new restrictive barrier;

5. Repeat this isometric contraction and stretch 3–5 times or until pelvic mobility returns; if successful, consider prescribing QUADRICEPS STRETCH.

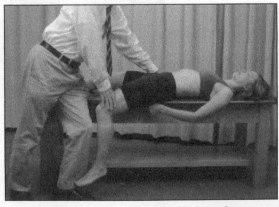

Muscle energy for left posterior innominate

QUADRICEPS STRETCH

1. Lie on your back with the involved leg hanging off the end of the bed or table;
2. Pull your other knee toward the chest;
3. Let the foot of the involved leg hang down as far as it can comfortably go;
4. Take a few deep breaths and stretch for 10–20 seconds;
5. Repeat for the other leg;
6. Do this stretch 2–4 times a day.

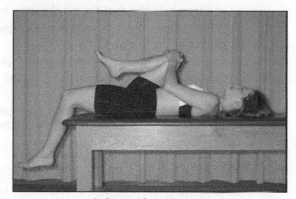

Left quadriceps stretch

POSTERIOR INNOMINATE THRUST—LATERAL RECUMBENT

INDICATIONS: Posterior innominate rotation associated with back pain, hip pain, short leg syndrome, and other problems.

RELATIVE CONTRAINDICATIONS: Acute lumbar sprain, undiagnosed radiculopathy, acute vertebral fracture, acute herniated or ruptured disc, or sacroiliac joint hypermobility.

TECHNIQUE:

1. Stand in front of the patient who is lying with the involved pelvis upward;

2. Flex the involved hip until movement is felt at the lumbosacral junction and then tuck that foot behind the other knee;

3. Rotate the back toward the table by lifting the table-side arm until you feel rotation at the lumbosacral junction;

4. Use your cephalad arm to stabilize the shoulder, place your other hand on the posterior aspect of the iliac crest, and lean over top of that hand;

5. Ask the patient to take a deep breath, and during exhalation slowly push the iliac crest toward the femur to take up the rotational slack;

6. At the end of exhalation, apply a short quick thrust with your arm and body onto the iliac crest toward the femur;

7. Recheck sacroiliac mobility or pelvis symmetry; if successful, consider prescribing SACROILIAC SELF-MOBILIZATION on p. 110 (in Chapter 5).

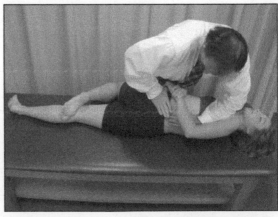

Lateral recumbent thrust for left posterior innominate

POSTERIOR INNOMINATE THRUST—SUPINE

INDICATIONS: Posterior innominate rotation or superior innominate shear associated with back pain, pelvis pain, hip pain, and other problems.

RELATIVE CONTRAINDICATIONS: Acute sacroiliac sprain, sacroiliac joint hypermobility, or hip or knee instability.

TECHNIQUE:

1. Stand at the foot of the table and grasp above the ankle with both hands above the malleoli;

2. Slightly abduct and internally rotate the leg;

3. Ask the patient to take a deep breath and during exhalation apply a firm and quick caudad tug down the leg;

4. Retest sacroiliac motion or pelvis symmetry; if successful, consider prescribing SACROILIAC SELF-MOBILIZATION on p. 110 (in Chapter 5).

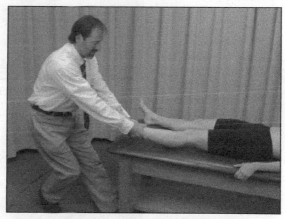

Traction tug for left posterior innominate rotation or superior innominate shear

PUBIC MUSCLE ENERGY/THRUST

INDICATIONS: Pubic symphysis compression or shear associated with pelvic pain, low back pain, and other problems.

RELATIVE CONTRAINDICATIONS: Acute pelvis fracture or post-partum.

TECHNIQUE (supine):

1. Grasp the outside of both knees that are flexed with feet flat on the table;

2. Ask the patient to push the knees apart for 3–5 seconds against your equal resistance;

3. Separate the knees by holding the inside of the knees and ask the patient to push the knees together for 3–5 seconds against your equal resistance;

4. Allow full relaxation and then repeat the isometric contraction 3–5 times, or until pubic mobilization occurs;

5. If needed, add a thrust to step 3 by applying a short and quick lateral push to overcome adduction contraction and further separate the knees;

6. Retest for pubic asymmetry; if successful, consider prescribing PUBIC SELF-MOBILIZATION.

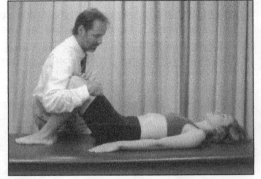

Abduction muscle energy

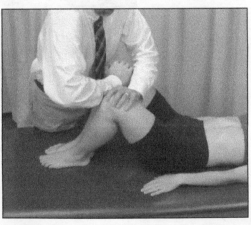

Adduction muscle energy/abduction thrust

PUBIC SELF-MOBILIZATION

1. Lie on your back with knees bent, feet on the floor, and head on a pillow or two;
2. Place your hands on the outside of the thighs;
3. Push your knees outward against resistance from your hands for 3–5 seconds;
4. Place a firm ball between the knees;
5. Push your knees inward against the ball for 3–5 seconds;
6. Repeat 1–3 times;
7. Do up to twice a day, if helpful.

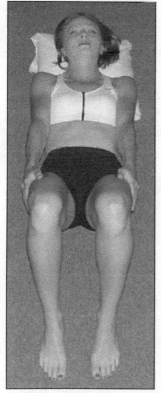

Abduction contraction

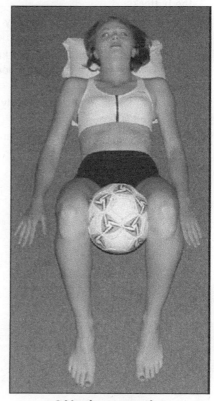

Adduction contraction

ILIUM INFLARE MUSCLE ENERGY

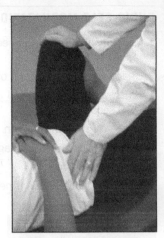

Muscle energy for left ilium inflare

INDICATIONS: Ilium inflare associated with back pain, pelvic pain, hip pain, and other problems.

RELATIVE CONTRAINDICATIONS: Acute pelvis fracture, sacroiliac joint inflammation, or severe hip arthritis.

TECHNIQUE (supine):

1. Stand on the opposite side of the inflare and flex the knee and hip, placing the foot on the table close to the buttocks;

2. Hold the opposite ASIS and laterally abduct the hip to the restrictive barrier;

3. Ask the patient to gently push the knee medially for 3–5 seconds against your equal resistance;

4. Allow full relaxation and then slowly laterally abduct the hip to a new restrictive barrier;

5. Repeat this isometric contraction and stretch 3–5 times or until motion returns;

6. Retest pelvis symmetry.

ILIUM OUTFLARE MUSCLE ENERGY

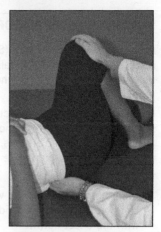

Muscle energy for right ilium outflare

INDICATIONS: Ilium outflare associated with back pain, pelvic pain, hip pain, and other problems.

RELATIVE CONTRAINDICATIONS: Acute pelvis fracture, sacroiliac joint inflammation, or severe hip arthritis.

TECHNIQUE (supine):

1. Stand on the side of the outflare and flex the knee and hip, placing the foot on the table close to the buttocks;

2. Pull the PSIS laterally and medially adduct the hip to the restrictive barrier;

3. Ask the patient to gently push the knee into external rotation for 3–5 seconds against your equal resistance;

4. Allow full relaxation and then slowly medially adduct the hip to a new restrictive barrier;

5. Repeat this isometric contraction and stretch 3–5 times, or until motion returns;

6. Retest pelvis symmetry.

SACROILIAC ARTICULATORY

INDICATIONS: Sacroiliac joint (SIJ) restriction related to back pain, pelvis pain, hip pain, and other problems.

RELATIVE CONTRAINDICATIONS: Acute sprain or fracture, SIJ hypermobility, SIJ inflammation, hip arthritis, deep venous thrombosis, premature labor.

TECHNIQUE (lateral Sims):

1. Stand behind the patient who is lying on the uninvolved side with the chest down;

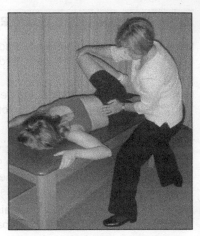

Flexion, abduction, and external rotation

2. Place the thenar eminence of your cephalad hand on the sacral base of the restricted SIJ and grasp the knee with your other hand;

3. Lean into the sacral base to stabilize the sacrum, have the patient take a deep breath and hold it, and slowly flex the hip to its restrictive barrier;

4. Slowly abduct and externally rotate the hip to its restrictive barrier;

5. Maintain the abduction barrier and slowly extend the hip fully;

6. Repeat as one smooth motion 3–5 times or until joint motion returns;

7. Retest sacroiliac motion; if successful, consider prescribing SACROILIAC SELF-MOBILIZATION on p. 110 (in Chapter 5).

REFERENCE

1. Adapted from Greenman PE. *Principles of Manual Medicine*, 2nd ed. Baltimore, MD: Williams & Wilkins; 1996.

5 Sacrum Diagnosis and Treatment

Diagnosis of Sacrum Somatic Dysfunction:
1. Screening tests
   Seated flexion test *p. 90*
   Sacrum palpation see *p. 91*
2. Sacrum motion tests
   Lumbosacral spring test *p. 92*
   Backward bending test *p. 92*
   Respiratory motion test *p. 93*
   Sacrum diagnosis using inherent motion *p. 94*
3. Sacrum somatic dysfunction diagnosis (Table 5-1) *p. 95*

Treatment of Sacrum Somatic Dysfunction:
1. OMT
   Sacrum counterstrain *p. 97*
   Mid-pole sacroiliac counterstrain *p. 98*
   Piriformis counterstrain *p. 99*
   Sacral-rocking/myofascial release *p. 101*
   Sacrum-balanced membranous tension *p. 102*
   Sacroiliac percussion vibrator *p. 103*
   Sacrum-facilitated oscillatory release *p. 104*
   Forward sacral torsion muscle energy *p. 105*
   Backward sacral torsion muscle energy *p. 106*
   Sacral extension muscle energy *p. 107*
   Sacral flexion muscle energy *p. 108*
   Unilateral sacral flexion thrust *p. 109*
2. Exercises
   Piriformis position of ease *p. 100*
   Piriformis stretch *p. 100*
   Sacroiliac self-mobilization *p. 110*
   Sacroiliac sidebending self-mobilization *p. 111*

89

Diagnosis

SCREENING TEST

Seated Flexion Test

1. Place your thumbs on the undersurface of the posterior superior iliac spines (PSIS) of the seated patient, taking care to keep both thumbs horizontal;

2. Ask the patient to bend forward with feet on the floor and allow your thumbs to follow PSIS movement, taking care to maintain both thumbs underneath the PSIS;

3. The side on which the PSIS stops moving superiorly the last is the side of sacrum restriction at the sacroiliac joint;

4. False positives: pelvis somatic dysfunction on same side.

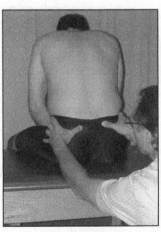

Seated flexion test

Sacrum Palpation

1. Stand to one side of the prone patient;
2. Palpate for tenderness at the following locations:
   a) **Sacrum tender points**
      i) sacral base on both sides and midline
      ii) middle sacrum on both sides and midline
      iii) lower sacrum on both sides and midline
   b) Sacrococcygeal junction;
   c) Tip of coccyx;
   d) **Mid-pole sacroiliac tender point**—inferior lateral angle of sacrum 1–2" inferior to the PSIS (see *p. 98*);
   e) **Piriformis tender point**—halfway between middle of sacral border and greater trochanter (see *p. 99*);
3. Sacral base levelness: Place your thumbs on the sacral base just medial to the PSIS and compare for anterior–posterior levelness;
4. Inferior lateral angle (ILA) levelness: Place your thumbs on the posterior surface and compare for anterior–posterior levelness or place your thumbs on the inferior surface and compare for superior–inferior levelness.

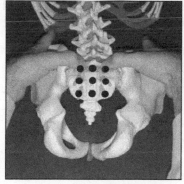

Sacral base palpation

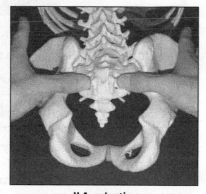

ILA palpation

SACRAL MOTION TESTS

Lumbosacral Spring Test

1. With the patient prone, use one or both palms to firmly push the lumbosacral junction in an anterior direction several times;
2. Negative (normal) test = ease of springing motion = sacral flexion ease or extension restriction;
3. Positive test = resistance to springing = sacral flexion restriction or extension ease.

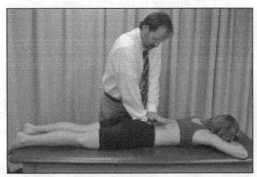

Lumbosacral spring test

Backward Bending Test (lumbosacral flexion test)

1. With the patient prone, place your thumbs on each side of the sacral base to identify asymmetry;
2. Ask the patient to place the elbows on the table and lift the upper back to induce relative sacral flexion;
3. Decreased sacral base asymmetry (negative test) indicates sacral flexion ease, extension restriction;
4. Positive test = increased sacral base asymmetry = sacral flexion restriction, extension ease.

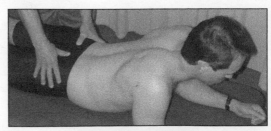

Backward bending test

Respiratory Motion Test

1. With the patient prone, let your hand rest gently on the sacrum with fingertips at sacral base and palm at coccyx;
2. Ask the patient to take a deep breath and follow the sacrum into anatomical extension with inhalation and anatomical flexion with exhalation;
3. Restriction of sacral extension indicates flexion ease;
4. Restriction of sacral flexion indicates extension ease.

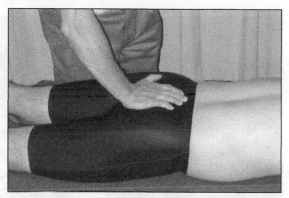

Respiratory motion testing of sacrum

Sacrum Diagnosis Using Inherent Motion*

1. With the patient supine, place your hand gently under the sacrum with fingertips at sacral base and the base of the palm just superior to the coccyx;
2. Let the hand relax by leaning onto your elbow;
3. Palpate craniosacral flexion (base posterior) and extension (base anterior);
4. Restricted craniosacral flexion indicates extension ease;
5. Restricted craniosacral extension indicates flexion ease.

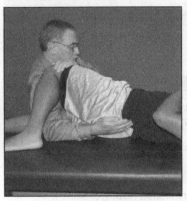
Hand positioning

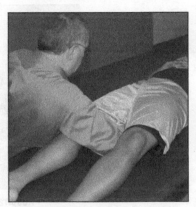
Palpation of flexion/extension

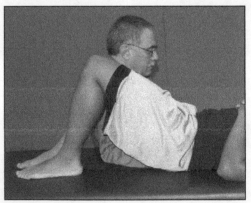
Alternate arm position

*The term *inherent motion* refers to a palpable cyclic pressure fluctuation variably referred to as cranial rhythmic impulse, craniosacral motion, entrainment, primary respiratory mechanism, pulse pressure fluctuation, and Traube–Hering–Mayer wave.

Table 5-1 | SACRUM SOMATIC DYSFUNCTION DIAGNOSIS

Diagnosis	Seated Flexion Test[a]	Sacral Base Levelness[b]	ILA Levelness	L5 Rotation[c]	Sacral Motion Testing[d]
Left-on-left torsion[e]	Right	Anterior right	Posterior left	Right	Extension restriction
Left-on-right torsion[e]	Left	Anterior right	Posterior left	Right	Flexion restriction
Right-on-right torsion[e]	Left	Anterior left	Posterior right	Left	Extension restriction
Right-on-left torsion[e]	Right	Anterior left	Posterior right	Left	Flexion restriction
Left unilateral flexion[f]	Left	Anterior left	Posterior left	–	Extension restriction
Left unilateral extension[f]	Left	Anterior right	Posterior right	–	Restriction
Right unilateral flexion[f]	Right	Anterior right	Posterior right	–	Extension restriction
Right unilateral extension[f]	Right	Anterior left	Posterior left	–	Flexion restriction

[a]With a sacral torsion, the seated flexion test is positive on the opposite side of the involved oblique axis.
[b]With a sacral torsion, the sacrum is rotated to the opposite side of the anterior sacral base.
[c]With a sacral torsion, L5 is rotated to the opposite side of sacral rotation. If L5 is rotated to the same side as the sacrum the dysfunction is termed a sacral rotation.
[d]Motion testing can be done with the lumbosacral spring test, backward-bending test, respiratory motion testing, or axis motion testing.
[e]Torsions are named for the direction on the axis: Left-on-left torsion = rotation left-on-a-left oblique axis.
[f]Also known as sacral shear.

95

KEY TO FIGURES IN TABLE 5-1: Findings for a left-on-left sacral torsion

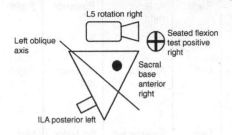

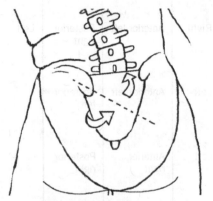

Sacrum rotation left on a left oblique axis (Drawing by William A. Kuchera, DO, FAAO)

Treatment

SACRUM COUNTERSTRAIN

INDICATIONS: Sacrum tender point associated with back pain, pelvic pain, and other problems.

RELATIVE CONTRAINDICATIONS: Acute sacral fracture, unable to lay prone.

TECHNIQUE (prone):

1. Locate the tender point on the posterior surface of the sacrum, labeling it 10/10;

2. Use your palm to push firmly into the sacrum as far from the tender point as possible, avoiding pressure on the coccyx;

3. Retest for tenderness;

4. Fine-tune this position with slightly more or less sacral pressure until tenderness is minimized to 0/10 if possible, but at most to 3/10;

5. Hold the position of maximum relief for 90 seconds, maintaining finger contact to monitor for tissue texture changes but reducing pressure;

6. Slowly remove sacral pressure and retest for tenderness with the same pressure as initial labeling.

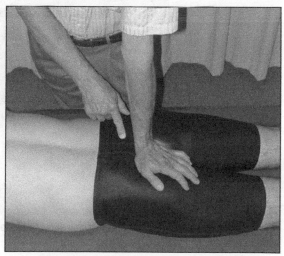

Sacrum tender point and treatment position

MID-POLE SACROILIAC COUNTERSTRAIN

INDICATIONS: Mid-pole sacroiliac tender point associated with back pain, pelvic pain, hip pain, and other problems.

RELATIVE CONTRAINDICATIONS: Severe hip arthritis, or deep venous thrombosis in involved leg.

TECHNIQUE (prone):

1. Locate the tender point by pushing medially onto the inferior lateral angle, labeling it 10/10;

2. Bend the knee on the tender point side and slightly abduct, flex, and externally rotate the hip until tenderness is minimized to 0/10 if possible, but at most to 3/10;

3. Hold this position of maximum relief for 90 seconds, maintaining finger contact to monitor for tissue texture changes but reducing pressure;

4. Slowly return the leg to the table and retest for tenderness with the same pressure as initial labeling.

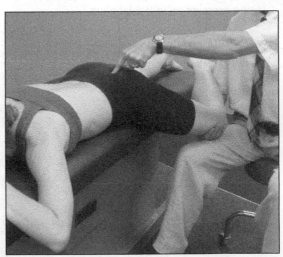

Mid-pole sacroiliac counterstrain

PIRIFORMIS COUNTERSTRAIN

INDICATIONS: Piriformis tender point associated with back pain, pelvic pain, hip pain, sciatic neuritis (see PIRIFORMIS MUSCLE AND SCIATIC NERVE), and other problems.

RELATIVE CONTRAINDICATIONS: Severe hip arthritis, deep venous thrombosis in involved leg, hip replacement, or history of hip dislocation.

TECHNIQUE (prone):

1. Locate the tender point in the mid-buttock halfway between the top of the greater trochanter and the mid-line of the sacrum, labeling it 10/10;

2. Bend the knee on the tender point side, flex the hip 90°, and abduct and externally rotate the hip until tenderness is minimized to 0/10 if possible, but at most to 3/10;

3. Hold this position of maximum relief for 90 seconds, maintaining finger contact to monitor for tissue texture changes but reducing pressure;

4. Slowly return the leg to the table and retest for tenderness with the same pressure as initial labeling; if successful, consider prescribing the PIRIFORMIS POSITION OF EASE and/or PIRIFORMIS STRETCH.

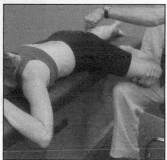

Piriformis counterstrain

PIRIFORMIS MUSCLE AND SCIATIC NERVE

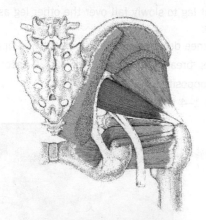

Sciatic nerve passes inferior to or through piriformis muscle

PIRIFORMIS POSITION OF EASE

1. Lie on your back with legs propped up on a chair or stool;
2. Cross your ankles with the foot on the side of back pain on top;
3. Let your knees fall apart;
4. If comfortable, take a few deep breaths and rest in this position for 2–5 minutes;
5. Slowly uncross your legs, bring them down, and roll to one side before getting up;
6. Use this position 2–4 times a day, or as needed for pain relief.

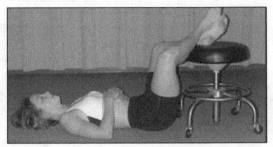

Piriformis position of ease

PIRIFORMIS STRETCH

1. Lie on your back and place one foot on top of the other knee;
2. Grasp the outside of the bent knee with your opposite hand;
3. Allow your bent leg to slowly fall over the other leg as far as it will comfortably go;
4. Pull the bent knee down toward the floor with the opposite hand;
5. Take a few deep breaths and stretch for 10–20 seconds;
6. Repeat to the opposite side;
7. Do this stretch 1–4 times a day.

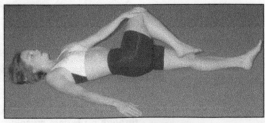

Piriformis stretch

SACRAL ROCKING/MYOFASCIAL RELEASE

INDICATIONS: Sacral restriction associated with back pain, pelvic pain, sciatic neuritis, constipation, diarrhea, dysmenorrhea, and other problems.

RELATIVE CONTRAINDICATIONS: Sacral fracture, sacroiliitis, premature labor, placenta previa, placental abruption, or bowel obstruction.

TECHNIQUE (prone, lateral):

1. Place your hands on the sacrum with the bottom hand pointing cephalad and your top hand pointing caudad;

2. Ask the patient to take a deep breath and encourage sacral extension during inhalation by pushing the sacral apex anteriorly;

3. During exhalation encourage sacral flexion by pushing the sacral base anteriorly;

4. Repeat 3–5 times;

5. Alternative technique using myofascial release:

   a) Evaluate flexion by moving the sacral fascia superiorly and extension by moving the sacral fascia inferiorly to determine directions of restriction and laxity;

   b) Indirect: Hold the sacral fascia in the position of laxity and follow any tissue release until completed;

   c) Direct: Hold the sacral fascia in the direction of restriction and apply steady force until tissue give is completed;

6. Retest sacral motion.

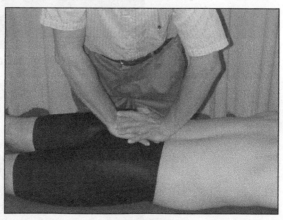

Sacral rocking

SACRUM BALANCED MEMBRANOUS TENSION

INDICATIONS: Restricted lumbosacral motion associated with back pain, pelvic pain, headache, and other problems.

CONTRAINDICATIONS: Acute sacrum fracture.

TECHNIQUE (supine):

1. Place one hand on the sacrum with fingertips at the base and palm at coccyx and your other hand across the lower lumbar spine;

2. Allow the sacral hand to relax by leaning onto your elbow;

3. Palpate craniosacral flexion (base posterior) and extension (base anterior), identifying directions of ease and restriction;

4. Use your hands and intention to exaggerate the direction of ease, resisting return to neutral until motion stops in a still point;

5. Maintain this position until motion returns and then gently follow it back to neutral before releasing pressure;

6. Reevaluate lumbosacral flexion and extension.

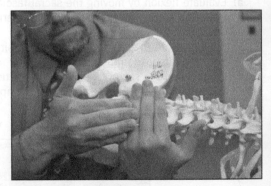

Hand positioning

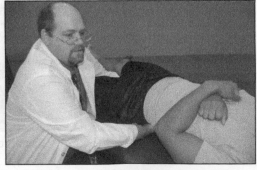

Sacrum balanced membranous tension

SACROILIAC PERCUSSION VIBRATOR

INDICATIONS: Restricted sacrum or pelvis motion associated with back pain, pelvic pain, and other problems.

RELATIVE CONTRAINDICATIONS: Acute fracture, sacroiliitis, undiagnosed radiculopathy, intrapelvic cancer, hip replacement, or pregnancy.

TECHNIQUE (lateral):

1. With the patient lying on the nonrestricted side with knees and hips flexed, place your monitoring hand over the greater trochanter and place the vibrating percussor pad lightly on the sacral base;

2. Adjust pad speed, pressure, and angle until vibrations are palpated as strong by the monitoring hand, avoiding pad bouncing;

3. Maintain contact until the force and rhythm of vibration returns to that of normal tissue;

4. Alternative technique:

   a) Allow the monitoring hand to be pulled toward the pad, resisting any other direction of hand pull;

   b) Maintain percussion until the monitoring hand is pushed away from the pad;

5. Slowly release the monitoring hand and the percussion vibrator and retest motion.

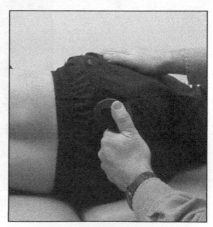

Sacroiliac percussion vibrator

SACRUM FACILITATED OSCILLATORY RELEASE

INDICATIONS: Sacral somatic dysfunction associated with back pain, pelvic pain, and other problems.

RELATIVE CONTRAINDICATIONS: Acute fracture or significant patient guarding.

TECHNIQUE (prone):

1. Place the heel of your cephalad hand on the lumbar or thoracic transverse processes and the heel of your other hand on the posterior prominence of the sacrum;

2. Localize as appropriate, using your radial or ulnar styloid process to make contact with a particular segment;

3. Initiate oscillatory motion of the trunk by rhythmically moving the cephalad hand right and left;

4. Direct your corrective force through the caudad hand against the most posterior portion of the sacrum;

5. Continue vertebral oscillation or modify its force until sacrum mobility improves.

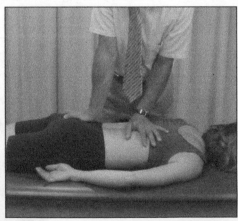

Sacrum facilitated oscillatory release

FORWARD SACRAL TORSION MUSCLE ENERGY

INDICATIONS: Forward sacral torsion or rotation (left on left, right on right) associated with back pain, pelvic pain, hip pain, and other problems.

RELATIVE CONTRAINDICATIONS: Acute sacroiliac sprain, acute sacrum fracture, severe knee arthritis, deep venous thrombosis, or premature labor.

TECHNIQUE (lateral Sims):

1. Sit or stand beside the patient who is lying on the axis side with the chest down on the table;

2. Flex the knees and hips until motion is felt at the lumbosacral junction, usually at least 90° hip flexion;

3. Allow the legs to hang down off the table with thighs supported by your leg or a pillow to avoid pressure from the table;

4. Monitor the anterior sacral base and ask the patient to push the feet toward the ceiling for 3–5 seconds against your equal resistance;

5. Allow full relaxation and then slowly move the legs toward the floor to a new restrictive barrier;

6. Repeat this isometric contraction and stretch 3–5 times, or until return of sacral mobility;

7. Retest sacroiliac motion or sacral symmetry.

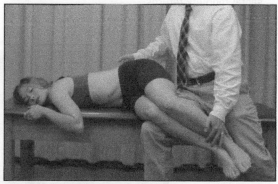

Muscle energy for right-on-right sacral torsion

BACKWARD SACRAL TORSION MUSCLE ENERGY

INDICATIONS: Backward sacral torsion or rotation (left on right, right on left) associated with back pain, pelvic pain, hip pain, and other problems.

RELATIVE CONTRAINDICATIONS: Acute sacroiliac sprain, acute sacrum fracture, severe hip arthritis, deep venous thrombosis, or premature labor.

TECHNIQUE (lateral recumbent):

1. Sit or stand in front of the patient who is lying on the axis side with the upper back on the table;

2. Extend the leg on the table until motion is felt at the lumbosacral junction;

3. Flex the top leg and place the foot behind the other knee;

4. Hold the shoulder to prevent the patient from rolling and allow the flexed knee to hang down off the table;

5. Ask the patient to push the flexed knee toward the ceiling for 3–5 seconds against your equal resistance;

6. Allow full relaxation and then slowly move the knee toward the floor to a new restrictive barrier;

7. Repeat this isometric contraction and stretch 3–5 times, or until sacral mobility returns;

8. Retest sacroiliac motion or sacral symmetry.

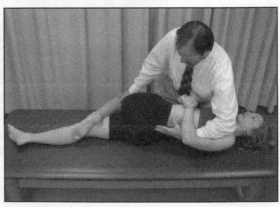

Muscle energy for left-on-right sacral torsion

SACRAL EXTENSION MUSCLE ENERGY

INDICATIONS: Unilateral or bilateral sacral extension associated with back pain, pelvis pain, hip pain, and other problems.

RELATIVE CONTRAINDICATIONS: Acute sacroiliac sprain, acute sacrum fracture, or premature labor.

TECHNIQUE (prone):

1. Stand facing the patient's feet on the side of the unilateral extension;

2. Place your thenar or hypothenar eminence on the involved sacral base and push it anteriorly and inferiorly by leaning into it. For a bilateral sacral extension push on both sides of the sacral base;

3. Use your other hand to slightly abduct and internally rotate the lower extremity on the involved side;

4. While the patient takes a deep breath, resist sacral extension during inhalation and push the sacrum into flexion during exhalation;

5. Repeat this isometric contraction and stretch 3–5 times, or until sacral mobility returns;

6. Retest sacroiliac motion or sacral symmetry.

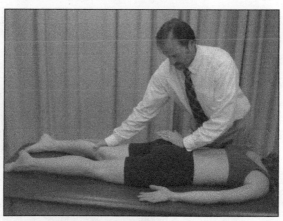

Muscle energy for left unilateral extension

SACRAL FLEXION MUSCLE ENERGY

INDICATIONS: Unilateral or bilateral sacral flexion associated with back pain, pelvis pain, hip pain, and other problems.

RELATIVE CONTRAINDICATIONS: Acute sacroiliac sprain, sacroiliac joint hypermobility, acute sacrum fracture, or premature labor.

TECHNIQUE (prone):

1. Stand facing the patient's head on the side of the unilateral flexion;

2. Place your thenar or hypothenar eminence on the involved inferior lateral angle and push it anteriorly and superiorly by leaning into it, avoiding pressure on the coccyx. For a bilateral sacral flexion push on both ILAs;

3. Use your other hand to slightly abduct and internally rotate the lower extremity on the involved side;

4. While the patient takes a deep breath, push the sacrum into extension during inhalation and resist sacral flexion during exhalation;

5. Repeat this isometric contraction and stretch 3–5 times, or until sacral mobility returns;

6. Retest sacroiliac motion or sacral symmetry.

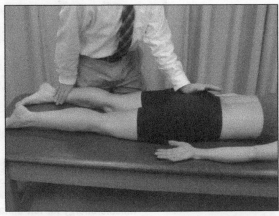

Muscle energy for left unilateral flexion

UNILATERAL SACRAL FLEXION THRUST

INDICATIONS: Unilateral sacral flexion (sacral shear) associated with back pain, pelvis pain, hip pain, and other problems.

RELATIVE CONTRAINDICATIONS: Acute sacroiliac sprain, acute sacrum fracture, hip or knee instability, or premature labor.

TECHNIQUE (supine or lateral):

1. Stabilize the inferior lateral angle (ILA) on the side of the unilateral flexion by placing a wedge on its inferior surface (supine one-person technique), or by having an assistant push the ILA superiorly and anteriorly (lateral two-person technique), avoiding pressure on the coccyx;

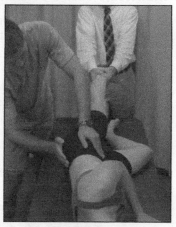

Two person thrust for left unilateral flexion

2. Standing at the foot of the table, grasp the ankle above the malleoli with both hands and slightly abduct and internally rotate the leg on the unilateral flexion side;

3. Ask the patient to take a deep breath and during exhalation apply a firm and quick tug down the leg;

4. Retest sacroiliac motion or sacral symmetry. If successful, consider prescribing the SACROILIAC SELF-MOBILIZATION and/or SACROILIAC SIDEBENDING SELF-MOBILIZATION.

SACROILIAC SELF-MOBILIZATION

1. Lie on your back and bend one leg up, grasping the knee with both hands. If the knee hurts, instead grasp the thigh behind the knee;

2. Pull the knee up toward your opposite shoulder as far as it will comfortably go;

3. Take a few deep breaths and with each exhalation pull the knee a little farther toward the opposite shoulder;

4. Use the opposite hand to pull the knee across your abdomen as you extend the leg;

5. Repeat for the other side;

6. Do up to twice a day, if helpful.

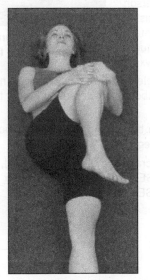
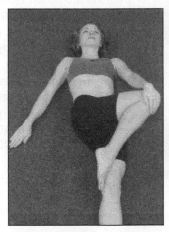

Flexion stretch   **Adduction with extension**

SACROILIAC SIDEBENDING SELF-MOBILIZATION

1. Lie on your back with knees bent and feet flat on the floor;

2. Reach your left hip outward and up toward your left shoulder as far as it will go;

3. Reach your right hip outward and up toward your right shoulder as far as it will go;

4. Repeat 1–3 times;

5. Do up to twice a day, if helpful.

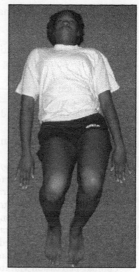

Sacroiliac sidebending self-mobilization

REFERENCE

1. Figure adapted with permission from Graham KE. *Outline of Muscle-Energy Techniques*. Tulsa, OK: Oklahoma College of Osteopathic Medicine and Surgery; 1985.

6 Lumbar Diagnosis and Treatment

Diagnosis of Lumbar Somatic Dysfunction

Treatment of Lumbar Somatic Dysfunction

Diagnosis

SCREENING TESTS

Hip Drop Test

1. Ask the standing patient to bend one knee and drop that hip, which induces lumbar sidebending away from the dropped hip;

2. Observe lumbar sidebending and amount of hip drop, which is normally $\geq 25°$;

3. Hip drop $<25°$ (positive test) indicates restricted lumbar sidebending toward the opposite side of the dropped hip.

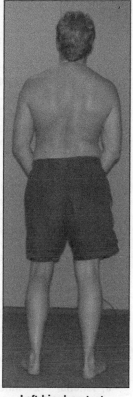

Left hip drop test (sidebending right)

Lumbosacral Fascial Rotation

1. With the patient supine, place your palms over the skin of the lateral pelvis and simultaneously lift one side while pushing the other side posteriorly to induce lumbosacral fascia rotation;

2. Repeat for the other direction to identify rotational restriction and laxity.

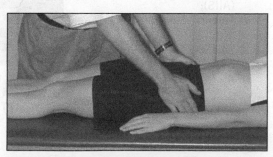

Lumbosacral fascial rotation

PALPATION

Lumbar Tender Points

1. Palpate for posterior lumbar tender points at the following locations:

   a) **Posterior T10–L5**—spinous processes or 1/2–1" lateral;

   b) **Posterior L3**—gluteal musculature halfway between posterior L4 and L5;

   c) **Posterior L4**—iliac crest in posterior axillary line;

   d) **Posterior L5** (upper pole L5)—superior surface of posterior superior iliac spine (PSIS) at insertion of iliolumbar ligament;

   e) **Lower pole L5**—inferior surface of the PSIS.

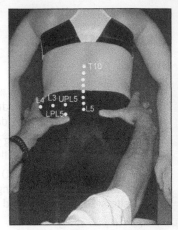

Posterior lumbar palpation (LPL5 shown)

2. Palpate for anterior lumbar tender points at the following locations:

   a) **Anterior T9**—1/2–1" superior to umbilicus;

   b) **Anterior T10**—1" below umbilicus;

   c) **Anterior T11**—2" below umbilicus;

   d) **Anterior T12**—inner aspect of iliac crest in mid-axillary line (not visible in photo);

   e) **Anterior L1**—1/2" medial to anterior superior iliac spine (ASIS);

   f) **Anterior L2**—medial surface of anterior inferior iliac spine (AIIS);

   g) **Anterior L3**—lateral surface of AIIS;

   h) **Anterior L4**—inferior surface of AIIS;

   i) **Anterior L5**—pubic ramus 1/2" lateral to pubic symphysis.

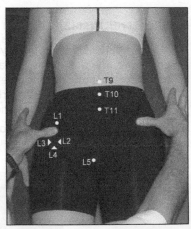

Anterior lumbar tender points (ASIS palpation shown, AT12 not shown)

Lumbar Rotation Testing—Seated

1. With the patient seated or prone, palpate the lumbar paraspinal area, comparing right and left sides for increased fullness;

2. Fullness may be due to muscle tension, edema, or vertebral rotation to that side;

3. Vertebral rotation multiple segments = neutral or type 1 somatic dysfunction with sidebending to opposite side;

4. Vertebral rotation single segment = nonneutral or type 2 somatic dysfunction with sidebending to same side—test flexion and extension;

5. Rotation worse in flexion = extension somatic dysfunction; rotation worse in extension = flexion somatic dysfunction.

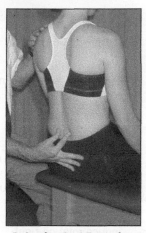

Palpation for L3 rotation

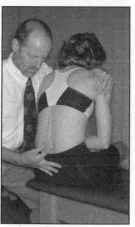

Flexion testing

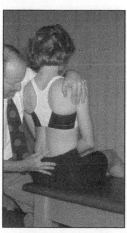

Extension testing

Lumbar Rotation Testing—Prone

1. With the patient prone or seated, place your thumbs on a lumbar vertebra's transverse processes located an inch lateral to the spinous process;

2. Push anteriorly on the right transverse process to induce rotation left; Push anteriorly on the left transverse process to induce rotation right;

3. Restricted rotation left = rotated right; Restricted rotation right = rotation left.

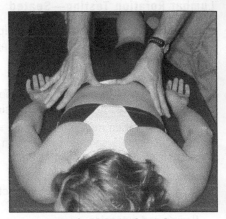

Testing L4 rotation left

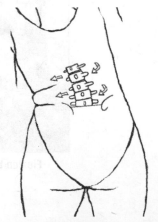

Neutral, sidebending left, rotation right (Drawing by William A. Kuchera, DO, FAAO)

Table 6-1 | THORACOLUMBAR SOMATIC DYSFUNCTION

Findings	Neutral or Type 1	Nonneutral or Type 2
Paraspinal fullness (rotation)	Multiple vertebrae	One vertebra
Sidebending	Opposite rotation	Same as rotation
Flexion or extension result	Minimal change	Fullness increases
Somatic dysfunction	N Rx Sy	F or E Rx Sx
Visceral association	Rare	Possible

Treatment

THORACOLUMBAR KNEADING/STRETCHING

INDICATIONS: Thoracic or lumbar paraspinal muscle tension associated with back pain, chest wall pain, and other problems.

RELATIVE CONTRAINDICATIONS: Acute lumbar strain and sprain, acute vertebral or rib fracture.

TECHNIQUE (prone):

1. Stand on the opposite side and place your cephalad palm on the tense muscle lateral to the spinous processes;

2. Grasp the ASIS on the side of tension with your caudad hand;

3. Slowly knead the tension by leaning into your cephalad hand with the arm straightened to push the muscle anteriorly and laterally, avoiding sliding over the skin;

4. Simultaneously stretch the tense muscle by slowly pulling your caudad hand posteriorly to lift the ASIS until resistance is felt;

5. Repeat simultaneous kneading and stretching until tension is reduced.

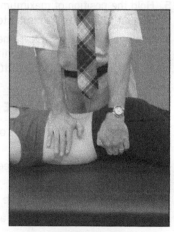

Thoracolumbar kneading/stretching

T10–L5 POSTERIOR COUNTERSTRAIN

INDICATIONS: Posterior T10–L5 tender point associated with back pain, pelvis pain, chest pain, and other problems.

RELATIVE CONTRAINDICATIONS: Acute fracture, hip dislocation, severe hip osteoarthritis.

TECHNIQUE (prone):

1. Locate the tender point, labeling it 10/10;

2. Stand on the opposite side and lift the thigh on the side of the tender point to extend the hip;

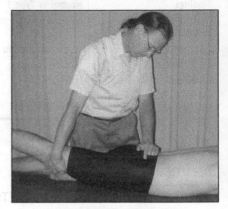

L3 posterior tender point and treatment position

3. Retest for tenderness;

4. Fine tune this position with slightly more hip extension, abduction, or adduction until tenderness is minimized to 0/10 if possible but at most 3/10;

5. Hold the position of maximum relief for 90 seconds, maintaining finger contact to monitor for tissue texture changes but reducing pressure;

6. Slowly and passively return the hip to neutral and retest for tenderness with the same pressure as initial labeling. If successful, consider prescribing LUMBAR POSITION OF EASE.

LUMBAR POSITION OF EASE

1. Lay face down with a pillow or two under your pelvis on the side of the back pain;

2. If comfortable, take a few deep breaths and rest in this position for 2–5 minutes;

3. Slowly roll to one side before getting up;

4. Use this position 2–4 times a day or as needed for pain relief.

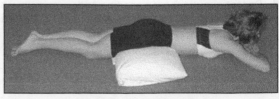

Lumbar position of ease

LOWER POLE L5 COUNTERSTRAIN

INDICATIONS: Lower pole L5 tender point associated with back pain, pelvic pain, hip pain, and other problems.

RELATIVE CONTRAINDICATIONS: Acute fracture, hip dislocation, and severe hip osteoarthritis.

TECHNIQUE (prone):

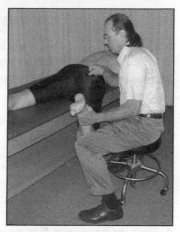

Lower pole L5 tender point and treatment position

1. Locate the tender point on the inferior aspect of the posterior superior iliac spine, labeling it 10/10;

2. Flex the hip and knee 90° and retest for tenderness;

3. Fine tune this position with slight hip adduction until tenderness is minimized to 0/10 if possible but at most 3/10;

4. Hold the position of maximum relief for 90 seconds, maintaining finger contact to monitor for tissue texture changes but reducing pressure;

5. Slowly and passively return the leg to the table and retest for tenderness with the same pressure as initial labeling.

T9–L5 ANTERIOR COUNTERSTRAIN

INDICATIONS: Anterior T9–L5 tender point associated with back pain, pelvic pain, chest wall pain, abdominal pain, and other problems.

RELATIVE CONTRAINDICATIONS: Acute lumbar fracture, acute lumbar strain and sprain.

TECHNIQUE (supine):

1. Stand beside the patient and locate the tender point, labeling it 10/10;

2. Passively flex the knees and hips 90° and retest for tenderness;

3. Fine tune this position with increased hip flexion and slight rotation or sidebending of the knees until tenderness is minimized to 0/10 if possible but at most 3/10;

4. Hold the position of maximum relief for 90 seconds, maintaining finger contact to monitor for tissue texture changes but reducing pressure;

5. Slowly and passively return the legs to the table and retest for tenderness with the same pressure as initial labeling.

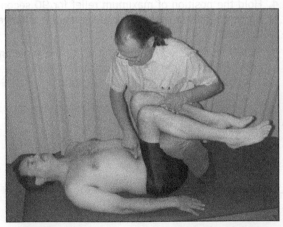

Anterior T10 tender point and treatment position

LUMBOSACRAL COMPRESSION/DECOMPRESSION

INDICATIONS: Lumbosacral tension related to back pain, sacroiliac pain, pelvic pain, and other problems.

RELATIVE CONTRAINDICATIONS: Acute lumbar or sacral fracture.

TECHNIQUE (prone or lateral):

1. Place one hand on the sacrum pointing caudad and the other hand on the lumbar spine pointing cephalad. Hands may also be pointed in the same direction;

2. Slowly pull your palms together to compress the lumbosacral fascia and then push your palms apart to decompress the lumbosacral fascia, determining directions of laxity and restriction;

3. Indirect: Move the lumbosacral fascia to its position of laxity and follow any tissue release until completed;

4. Direct: Move the lumbosacral fascia into its restriction and apply steady force until tissue give is completed;

5. Retest lumbosacral compression and decompression.

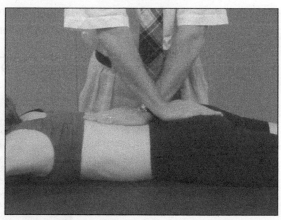

Lumbosacral compression/decompression

LUMBAR SOFT TISSUE-FACILITATED POSITIONAL RELEASE[1]

INDICATIONS: Lumbar paraspinal tension associated with back pain, pelvic pain, hip pain, and other problems.

RELATIVE CONTRAINDICATIONS: Acute lumbar fracture, severe hip arthritis.

TECHNIQUE (prone):

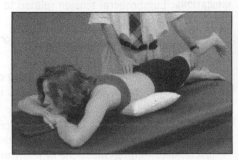

Lumbar soft tissue-facilitated positional release

1. Place a pillow under the abdomen to decrease lumbar lordosis;

2. Stand on the side of paraspinal tension, palpate the tension with your cephalad hand, and grasp the outside of the opposite distal thigh with your other hand;

3. Extend and adduct the leg until tension is reduced;

4. Hold this position for 3–5 seconds until tension release is completed;

5. Slowly lower the leg to the table and retest for tension.

LUMBAR FLEXION-FACILITATED POSITIONAL RELEASE[1]

INDICATIONS: Lumbar flexion somatic dysfunction associated with back pain and other problems.

RELATIVE CONTRAINDICATIONS: Severe hip arthritis.

TECHNIQUE (prone):

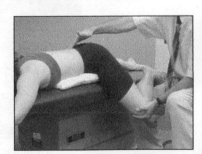

FPR for L5 FRS left

1. Place a pillow under the abdomen to decrease lumbar lordosis;

2. Sit on the side of lumbar rotation and palpate the paraspinal tension;

3. Flex the hip on the side of lumbar rotation by dropping the knee off the table until paraspinal tension decreases;

4. Add compression by lifting the knee or traction by letting the knee drop to further reduce paraspinal tension;

5. Hold this position for 3–5 seconds until tension release is completed and slowly return the leg to the table;

6. Remove the pillow and retest lumbar rotation.

LUMBAR EXTENSION-FACILITATED POSITIONAL RELEASE[1]

INDICATIONS: Lumbar extension somatic dysfunction associated with back pain and other problems.

RELATIVE CONTRAINDICATIONS: Severe hip arthritis.

TECHNIQUE (prone):

1. Position the patient with the hip on the side of lumbar rotation close to the edge of the table;
2. Place a pillow under the abdomen to decrease lumbar lordosis and another pillow between the mid-thigh and table;
3. Sit on the side of lumbar rotation and palpate the paraspinal tension;
4. Abduct the leg to create lumbar side bending to the side of lumbar rotation;
5. Hold the ankle and internally rotate the lower leg until motion is felt at the dysfunctional segment;
6. Push the leg downward to flex the hip until motion is felt at the dysfunctional segment;
7. Hold this position for 3–5 seconds until tension release is completed and slowly return the leg to the table;
8. Remove the pillows and retest lumbar rotation.

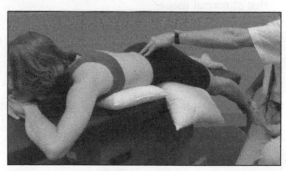

FPR for L5 ERS left

LUMBAR PERCUSSION VIBRATOR

INDICATIONS: Lumbar somatic dysfunction associated with back pain and other problems.

RELATIVE CONTRAINDICATIONS: Acute fracture, undiagnosed radiculopathy, lumbar or intrapelvic cancer, hip replacement, and pregnancy.

TECHNIQUE (lateral):

1. With the patient lying on the nonrestricted side with knees and hips flexed, place your monitoring hand over the greater trochanter;

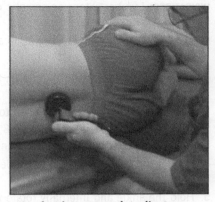

Lumbar percussion vibrator

2. Place the vibrating percussion pad lightly on the involved lumbar spinous processes perpendicular to the surface avoiding pad bouncing;

3. Alter pad speed, pressure, and angle until vibrations are palpated as strong by the monitoring hand;

4. Maintain contact until the force and rhythm of vibration returns to that of normal tissue;

5. Alternative technique:

   a) Allow the monitoring hand to be pulled toward the pad, resisting any other direction of hand pull;

   b) Maintain percussion until the monitoring hand is pushed away from the pad;

6. Slowly release the monitoring hand and the percussion vibrator and retest tissue texture or motion.

THORACOLUMBAR-FACILITATED OSCILLATORY RELEASE

INDICATIONS: Lumbar or thoracic somatic dysfunction associated with back pain, chest wall pain, or other problems.

RELATIVE CONTRAINDICATIONS: Acute fracture, significant patient guarding.

TECHNIQUE (prone):

1. Place one hand on the sacrum and the heel of your other hand over the posterior transverse processes or ribs;

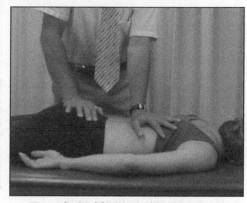

Thoracic-facilitated oscillatory release

2. Localize as appropriate using your radial or ulnar styloid process to make contact with a particular segment;

3. Initiate oscillatory motion of the pelvis by rhythmically moving your sacral hand right and left;

4. Add corrective force through your cephalad hand onto the transverse processes or ribs;

5. Continue pelvic oscillation or modify its force until you feel tension is reduced or mobility is improved.

LUMBAR SEATED FACET RELEASE

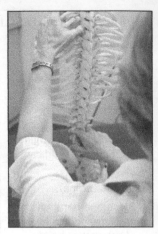
Hand positioning

INDICATIONS: Restricted lumbar movement associated with back pain, pelvic pain, and other problems.

RELATIVE CONTRAINDICATIONS: Joint inflammation, joint hypermobility, acute sprain, acute fracture, vertebral cancer, and undiagnosed lumbosacral radiculopathy.

TECHNIQUE:

1. Stand or sit behind the patient and have him or her markedly increase lumbar lordosis so that the shoulders are balanced over the pelvis;

2. Place a knuckle or finger on the inferior facet of the locked open or closed facet group;

3. Place your other hand on the shoulder and gently compress inferiorly while extending the area to be treated, keeping the shoulders balanced over the pelvis. Repeat for the other shoulder to determine the side of facet restriction;

4. Test the side of facet restriction for the position of greatest restriction by gentle compression and recoil on the shoulder to close and open the locked facet;

5. Hold the patient in the position of greatest restriction and gently induce a small amount of additional compression or traction through the shoulder to induce glide of the facet, thereby releasing the restriction;

6. Retest lumbar motion.

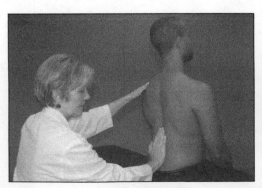
Initial position

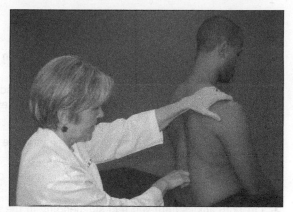

Testing right facet

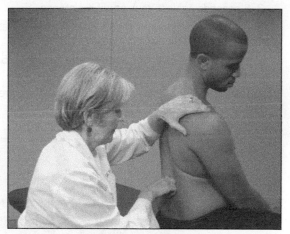

Right facet compression

LUMBAR MUSCLE ENERGY—LATERAL

INDICATIONS: Restricted multisegment lumbar rotation associated with back pain, scoliosis, and other problems.

RELATIVE CONTRAINDICATIONS: Acute lumbar sprain, undiagnosed radiculopathy, acute vertebral fracture, and vertebral cancer or infection.

TECHNIQUE:

1. Stand in front of the patient who is lying with the vertebral rotation side up;
2. Flex the hips until you feel motion in the middle of the restricted segments;
3. Lift both ankles until you feel sidebending in the middle of the restricted segments;
4. Ask the patient to push the ankles down toward the table for 3–5 seconds against your equal resistance;
5. Allow full relaxation and then slowly lift the ankles to a new lumbar sidebending restrictive barrier;
6. Repeat this isometric contraction and stretch 3–5 times or until lumbar mobility returns;
7. Retest lumbar rotation. If successful, consider prescribing LUMBAR EXTENSOR STRETCH.

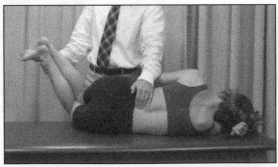

Muscle energy for L1–5 N R left S right

LUMBAR MUSCLE ENERGY—LATERAL RECUMBENT

INDICATIONS: Restricted lumbar rotation associated with back pain, scoliosis, and other problems.

RELATIVE CONTRAINDICATIONS: Acute lumbar sprain, undiagnosed radiculopathy, acute vertebral fracture, and vertebral cancer or infection.

TECHNIQUE:

1. Stand in front of the patient who is lying with the side of lumbar rotation toward the table;
2. Flex the upward hip until you feel motion at the restricted segment and tuck the foot behind the other knee;
3. Rotate the back toward the table by pushing the upward shoulder posteriorly and lifting the table-side arm and shoulder until you feel rotation at the restricted segment;
4. Place your forearm across the buttock, lean over top of that arm, and use your other arm to stabilize the patient's shoulder, taking care not to push into the ribs or breast;
5. Ask the patient to push the pelvis backward for 3–5 seconds against your equal resistance;
6. Allow full relaxation and then slowly move the pelvis anteromedially to a new lumbar rotation restrictive barrier;
7. Repeat 3–5 times or until lumbar mobility returns;
8. Retest lumbar rotation. If successful, consider prescribing LUMBAR EXTENSOR STRETCH.

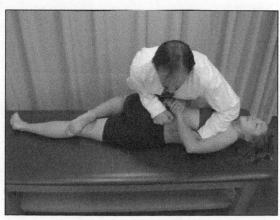

Muscle energy for L3 rotated right

LUMBAR EXTENSOR STRETCH

1. Lie on your back and grasp both knees with your hands. If knee pain occurs, instead grasp the thighs behind the knees;
2. Use your arms to slowly pull the knees toward the chest as far as they will comfortably go;
3. Take a few deep breaths and stretch for 10–20 seconds;
4. Do this stretch 1–4 times a day.

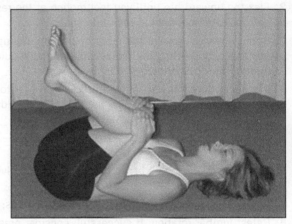

Lumbar extensor stretch

THORACOLUMBAR MUSCLE ENERGY/THRUST—SEATED

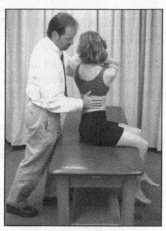

ME for L1–5 N R right S left

INDICATIONS: Restricted lumbar or thoracic rotation associated with back pain, scoliosis, and other problems.

RELATIVE CONTRAINDICATIONS: Acute lumbar sprain, joint hypermobility, undiagnosed radiculopathy, acute vertebral fracture, and vertebral cancer or infection.

TECHNIQUE:

1. Standing behind the seated patient, place your thenar eminence on the posterior transverse process(es);

2. Reach across the upper chest with your other hand and arm to control the patient's shoulders and trunk;

3. Move the trunk into the rotation, sidebending, and flexion–extension restrictive barriers until you feel movement at the restricted segment(s);

4. Ask the patient to straighten the trunk and/or shoulders for 3–5 seconds against your equal resistance;

5. Allow full relaxation and then slowly move the trunk to new restrictive barriers as you push anterior into the posterior transverse process(es);

6. Repeat this isometric contraction and stretch 3–5 times or until lumbar mobility returns;

7. Add a thrust if needed by a short and quick anterior push into the posterior transverse process(es) as you simultaneously move the trunk into its restrictive barriers;

8. Retest lumbar rotation. If successful, consider prescribing LUMBAR SELF-MOBILIZATION or THORACOLUMBAR STRETCH/SELF-MOBILIZATION.

LUMBOSACRAL ARTICULATORY/ THRUST—SUPINE

INDICATIONS: Restricted lumbar rotation or sacroiliac joint mobility associated with back pain, pelvic pain, and other problems.

RELATIVE CONTRAINDICATIONS: Joint inflammation, joint hypermobility, acute sprain, acute fracture, vertebral cancer, undiagnosed lumbosacral radiculopathy.

TECHNIQUE (supine):

1. Ask the patient to interlock his or her fingers behind the head;

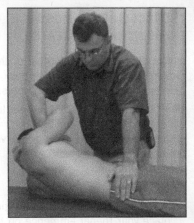

Lumbosacral articulatory/thrust (OB roll)

2. Stand to one side of the patient, use the palm of your caudad hand to hold the opposite anterior superior iliac spine (ASIS), and reach your cephalad hand over and through the patient's opposite elbow, placing the back of your hand on the sternum;

3. Lean into the ASIS and slowly pull the patient's arm toward you until reaching a rotation and flexion restrictive barrier;

4. If needed, apply a short and quick thrust posteriorly into the ASIS;

5. Retest lumbar rotation or sacroiliac mobility. If successful, consider prescribing LUMBAR SELF-MOBILIZATION or THORACOLUMBAR STRETCH/SELF-MOBILIZATION.

LUMBAR THRUST—LATERAL RECUMBENT (LUMBAR ROLL)

INDICATIONS: Restricted lumbar rotation associated with back pain, scoliosis, and other problems.

RELATIVE CONTRAINDICATIONS: Acute lumbar sprain, lumbar joint hypermobility, undiagnosed radiculopathy, acute vertebral fracture, acute herniated or ruptured disc, and vertebral cancer or infection.

TECHNIQUE:

1. Stand in front of the patient who is lying on the side of lumbar rotation;
2. Flex the upward hip until you feel motion at the restricted segment and then tuck the patient's foot behind the other knee;
3. Rotate the back toward the table by lifting the table-side arm until you feel rotation at the restricted segment;
4. Use your cephalad arm to stabilize the shoulder, place your other forearm across the buttock, and lean over top of that arm;
5. Ask the patient to take a deep breath and during exhalation slowly push the pelvis anteromedially to take up the rotational slack;
6. At the end of exhalation apply a short quick thrust with your arm and body onto the pelvis in an anteromedial direction;
7. Retest lumbar rotation. If successful, consider prescribing LUMBAR SELF-MOBILIZATION or THORACOLUMBAR STRETCH/ SELF-MOBILIZATION.

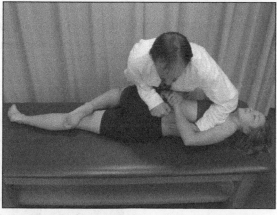

Lateral recumbent thrust for L3 rotated right

LUMBAR SELF-MOBILIZATION[2]

1. Lie on your back with knees bent, feet on the floor, and arms outstretched;
2. Drape one knee over the other and allow the legs to fall to the floor while keeping the shoulders down;
3. Repeat to the other side;
4. Do up to twice a day if helpful.

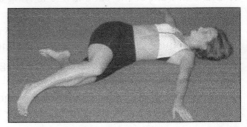

Lumbar self-mobilization

THORACOLUMBAR STRETCH/SELF-MOBILIZATION[2]

1. Sit with your legs straight and hands on the floor behind you;
2. Bend one knee and place the opposite arm against the outside of the bent leg;
3. Slowly turn your trunk toward the bent leg as far as it will comfortably go while pushing the arm into the leg;
4. Take a few deep breaths and stretch for 10–20 seconds;
5. For mobilization, add a short quick push of the arm into the leg to twist the trunk slightly farther;
6. Repeat to the other side;
7. Stretch 1–4 times a day and mobilize up to twice a day.

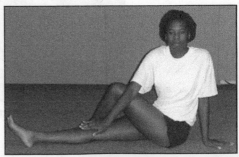

Thoracolumbar stretch/self-mobilization

REFERENCES

1. Adapted from Schiowitz S, DiGiovanna EL, Dowling DJ. Facilitated positional release [Chapter 64]. In: Ward RC, ed. *Foundations for Osteopathic Medicine.* 2nd ed. Philadelphia, PA: Lippincott Williams & Wilkins; 2003.

2. Adapted from Kirk CE. *Biodynamics of Self-Administered Manipulation. 1977 AAO Yearbook.* Colorado Springs, CO: American Academy of Osteopathy; 1979.

7 Thoracic Diagnosis and Treatment

Diagnosis of Thoracic Somatic Dysfunction
1. Screening: Acromion drop test *p. 137*
2. Thoracic tender points *p. 138*
3. Thoracic motion testing
   Thoracic rotation—seated *p. 139*
   Thoracic rotation—prone *p. 140*
   Thoracic inlet diagnosis using inherent motion *p. 141*
4. Thoracic somatic dysfunction (Table 7-1) *p. 142*

Treatment of Thoracic Somatic Dysfunction
1. OMT
   Thoracolumbar kneading *p. 142*
   Posterior T1–T9 midline counterstrain *p. 143*
   Posterior T1–T9 lateral counterstrain *p. 144*
   Anterior T1–T8 counterstrain *p. 145*
   Thoracolumbar myofascial release *p. 146*
   Cervicothoracic myofascial release *p. 147*
   Cervicothoracic myofascial release—seated *p. 148*
   Thoracic outlet direct myofascial release *p. 149*
   Thoracic myofascial release *p. 151*
   Thoracic extension-facilitated positional release *p. 152*
   Thoracic flexion-facilitated positional release *p. 153*
   Sternum ligamentous articular strain *p. 154*
   Thoracic percussion vibrator *p. 155*
   Thoracic-seated facet release *p. 156*
   Upper thoracic-seated facet release *p. 157*
   Thoracic muscle energy/thrust—seated *p. 159*
   Thoracic/rib articulatory—supine *p. 161*
   Thoracic thrust—prone *p. 161*
   Thoracic/rib thrust—supine *p. 162*
2. Exercises
   Posterior thoracic position of ease *p. 145*
   Anterior thoracic position of ease *p. 146*
   Thoracic flexion/extension stretch *p. 160*
   Thoracic/rib self-mobilization—supine *p. 163*
   Thoracic/rib thrust—seated *p. 163*
   Thoracic self-mobilization—kneeling *p. 164*
   Thoracic self-mobilization—standing *p. 165*

Diagnosis

ACROMION DROP TEST (thoracic sidebending)

1. Stand behind the seated patient and stabilize the head and shoulder with one arm;

2. Place your other hand across the acromion with your arm pointing inferiorly and medially;

3. Push the shoulder inferiorly and medially to test thoracic sidebending and repeat for the other side;

4. Resistance compared to the other side or acromion drop less than 20° indicates restricted thoracic sidebending to that side.

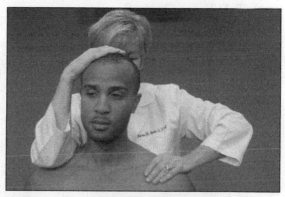

Testing left thoracic sidebending

THORACIC TENDER POINTS

1. Palpate for posterior thoracic tender points at the following locations:
   a) **Posterior T1–T9**—spinous process or 1/2" lateral;
   b) **Posterior T10–T12**—see *Chapter 8.*

2. Palpate for anterior thoracic tender points at the following locations:
   a) **T1**—sternal notch pushing inferiorly;
   b) **T2**—middle of manubrium;
   c) **T3–T4**—sternum at level of corresponding rib insertion;
   d) **T5**—1" above xiphisternal junction or at rib 5 cartilage;
   e) **T6**—xiphisternal junction or at rib 6 cartilage;
   f) **T7**—tip of xiphoid process or at rib 7 cartilage;
   g) **T8**—1.5" below xiphoid process or at chondral mass;
   h) **T9–T12**—see *Chapter 8.*

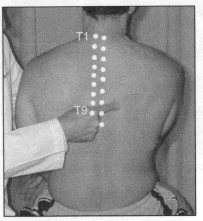

**Posterior thoracic tender points
(only midline and left
points illustrated)**

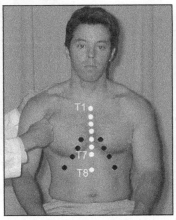

**Anterior thoracic tender points
(pectoralis minor
palpation shown)**

THORACIC MOTION TESTING

Thoracic Rotation—Seated

1. With the patient seated or prone, palpate the thoracic paraspinal area, comparing right and left sides for increased fullness and resistance to anterior pressure;

2. Fullness may be due to muscle tension, edema, or vertebral rotation to that side;

3. Vertebral rotation multiple segments = neutral or type 1 somatic dysfunction with sidebending to the opposite side;

4. Vertebral rotation single segment = nonneutral or type 2 somatic dysfunction with sidebending to the same side: test flexion and extension;

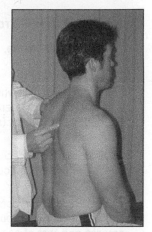

Palpation for T5 rotation

5. Induces passive flexion and extension as follows:

    T1–6—flex and extend the head;
    T7–12—flex and extend the trunk (see *Chapter 8*);

6. Increased tension with flexion = extension somatic dysfunction; increased tension with extension = flexion somatic dysfunction.

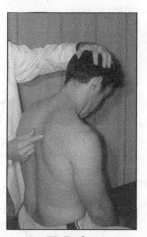

T5 flexion

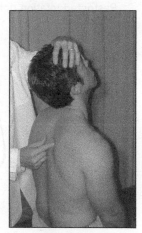

T5 extension

Thoracic Rotation—Prone

1. With the patient prone, place your thumbs on a thoracic vertebra's transverse processes which are located 1/2–1" lateral to the midline as follows (rule of threes):

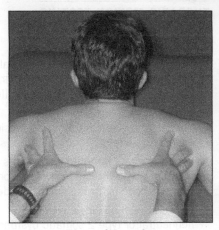

T6 rotation testing

T1–3—transverse processes directly lateral to spinous process;

T4–6—transverse processes halfway between spinous process and that of segment above;

T6–9—transverse processes directly lateral to spinous process of segment above;

T10–12—transverse processes return directly to lateral spinous process;

2. Push anteriorly on the right transverse process to induce rotation left;

   Push anteriorly on the left transverse process to induce rotation right;

3. Restricted rotation left = rotated right;

   Restricted rotation right = rotation left.

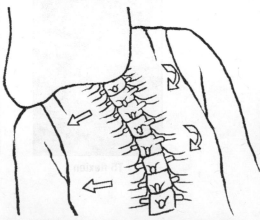

Neutral, sidebending left, and rotation right (Drawing by William A. Kuchera, DO, FAAO)

Thoracic Inlet Diagnosis Using Inherent Motion*

1. With the patient supine, place your hands gently over the top of the shoulders with fingertips along clavicles and thumbs on posterior upper trapezius muscles;

2. Palpate inherent flexion/external rotation and extension/internal rotation to identify restricted motion;

   a) Restricted bilateral flexion/external rotation indicates inherent extension;

   b) Restricted unilateral flexion indicates thoracic inlet sidebending or depressed first rib;

   c) Restricted unilateral external rotation indicates upper extremity internal rotation;

   d) Restricted bilateral extension/internal rotation indicates inherent flexion;

   e) Restricted unilateral extension indicates elevated first rib;

   f) Restricted unilateral internal rotation indicates upper extremity external rotation;

3. If related to the patient problem, treat the restriction with myofascial release, balanced membranous tension, or other techniques.

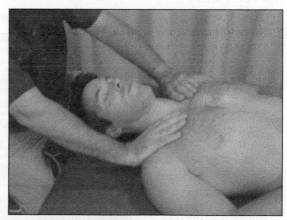

Palpation for thoracic inlet inherent motion

---

*The term inherent motion refers to a palpable cyclic pressure fluctuation variably referred to as cranial rhythmic impulse, craniosacral motion, entrainment, primary respiratory mechanism, pulse pressure fluctuation, and Traube–Hering–Mayer wave.

Table 7-1 I THORACIC SOMATIC DYSFUNCTION

Findings	Neutral or Type 1	Nonneutral or Type 2
Paraspinal fullness (rotation)	Multiple vertebrae	One vertebra
Sidebending	Opposite rotation	Same as rotation
Flexion or extension result	Minimal change	Fullness increases
Somatic dysfunction	N Rx Sy	F or E Rx Sx
Visceral association	Rare	Possible

Treatment

THORACOLUMBAR KNEADING

INDICATIONS: Thoracic or lumbar paraspinal muscle tension associated with back pain, chest wall pain, and other problems.

RELATIVE CONTRAINDICATIONS: Acute vertebral or rib fracture.

TECHNIQUE (lateral):

1. Stand facing the patient who is lying on the opposite side of paraspinal muscle tension;

2. Drape the patient's arm over your forearm to move the scapula away from the spine;

3. Grasp the tense muscle with the fingertips of one or both hands;

4. Slowly lean backward to pull the tense muscle laterally, avoiding sliding over the skin;

5. Repeat kneading until tension is reduced.

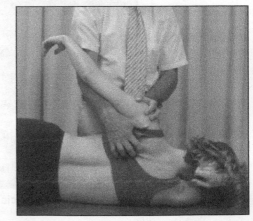

Thoracic kneading

POSTERIOR T1–T9 MIDLINE COUNTERSTRAIN

INDICATIONS: Midline posterior T1–T9 tender point associated with back pain, chest pain, neck pain, headache, and other problems.

RELATIVE CONTRAINDICATIONS: Acute fracture.

TECHNIQUE (prone):

1. Locate the tender point by pushing anteriorly into the spinous process, labeling it 10/10;

2. Have the patient cross their wrists in front of them and intertwine their fingers with palms facing each other;

3. Extend the upper thoracic spine by cupping the patient's wrists and gently lifting them, making sure not to extend the cervical spine;

4. Retest for tenderness and fine-tune this position with slightly more or less extension until tenderness is minimized to 0/10 if possible but at most 3/10;

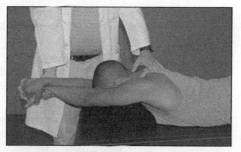

PT5 midline counterstrain, prone

5. Hold the position of maximum relief for 90 seconds, maintaining finger contact to monitor for tissue texture changes but reducing pressure;

6. Slowly and passively return the arms to the table and retest for tenderness with the same pressure as initial labeling;

7. Alternative position: Stand in front of the seated patient, place their hands over your shoulder, and extend the spine by pulling the upper back toward you.

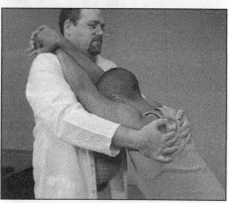

PT4 midline counterstrain, seated

POSTERIOR T1–T9 LATERAL COUNTERSTRAIN

INDICATIONS: Lateral posterior T1–T9 tender point associated with back pain, chest pain, shoulder pain, neck pain, headache, and other problems.

RELATIVE CONTRAINDICATIONS: Acute fracture, shoulder dislocation.

TECHNIQUE (prone):

1. Locate the tender point lateral to the spinous process, labeling it 10/10;

2. Lift the shoulder on the side of the tender point posteriorly toward the point and retest for tenderness;

3. Fine tune this position with slightly more or less shoulder lift until tenderness is minimized to 0/10 if possible but at most 3/10;

4. Hold the position of maximum relief for 90 seconds, maintaining finger contact to monitor for tissue texture changes but reducing pressure;

5. Slowly and passively return the shoulder to neutral and retest for tenderness with the same pressure as initial labeling. If successful, consider prescribing POSTERIOR THORACIC POSITION OF EASE.

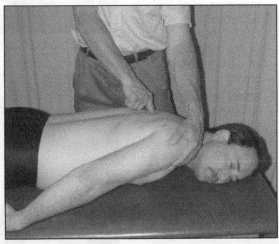

Counterstrain for right lateral PT5

POSTERIOR THORACIC POSITION OF EASE

1. Lay face down with a pillow or two under your shoulder on the side of back pain;

2. Turn your head to the side of back pain and allow it to rest on the pillow;

3. If back pain is reduced, take a few deep breaths and rest in this position for 2–5 minutes;

4. Repeat 2–4 times a day or as needed for pain relief.

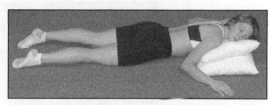

Posterior thoracic position of ease

ANTERIOR T1–T8 COUNTERSTRAIN

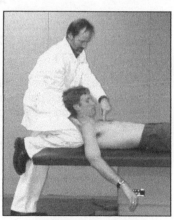

INDICATIONS: Anterior T1–T8 tender point associated with back pain, chest wall pain, and other problems.

RELATIVE CONTRAINDICATIONS: Acute thoracic or rib fracture, acute cervical fracture, or dislocation.

TECHNIQUE (supine):

1. Stand at the head of the table and locate the tender point, labeling it 10/10;

2. Flex the neck and upper back until tenderness is reduced, supporting the patient in this position with your arm, thigh, or abdomen;

AT4 tender point and treatment position

3. Retest for tenderness and fine tune this position with slightly more or less flexion until tenderness is minimized to 0/10 if possible but at most 3/10;

4. Hold the position of maximum relief for 90 seconds, maintaining finger contact to monitor for tissue texture changes but reducing pressure;

5. Slowly and passively return the patient to neutral and retest for tenderness with the same pressure as initial labeling. If successful, consider prescribing ANTERIOR THORACIC POSITION OF EASE.

ANTERIOR THORACIC POSITION OF EASE

1. Lie on your back with 2–3 pillows under the head;
2. If chest pain is reduced take a few deep breaths and rest in this position for 2–5 minutes. If pain is not reduced try adding or removing a pillow;
3. Repeat 2–4 times a day or as needed for pain relief.

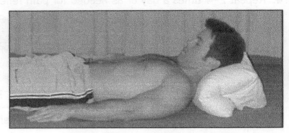

Anterior thoracic position of ease

THORACOLUMBAR MYOFASCIAL RELEASE (DIAPHRAGM, THORACIC OUTLET)

INDICATIONS: Restricted thoracolumbar rotation related to back pain, chest wall pain, edema, shortness of breath, and other problems.

RELATIVE CONTRAINDICATIONS: Acute costochondral subluxation.

TECHNIQUE (supine or prone):

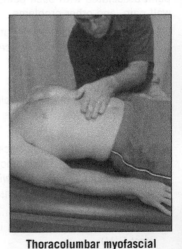

Thoracolumbar myofascial release

1. Place one hand across the chondral masses of the lower ribs and your other hand across the thoracolumbar spinous processes. Alternatively, place a hand on either side of the lower rib cage;
2. Indirect: Gently compress your hands together or rotate the fascia under your hands to the position of laxity, maintaining fascial laxity and following any tissue release until completed;
3. Direct: Gently move the thoracolumbar fascia into its superior–inferior, rotation, and sidebending restrictions and apply steady force until tissue give is completed;
4. Retest thoracolumbar rotation.

CERVICOTHORACIC MYOFASCIAL RELEASE (THORACIC INLET)

INDICATIONS: Restricted cervicothoracic rotation related to neck pain, headache, back pain, chest wall pain, edema, shortness of breath, and other problems.

RELATIVE CONTRAINDICATIONS: Acute clavicle fracture.

TECHNIQUE (supine):

1. Sit at the head of the table and place your hands across the top of the shoulders with fingertips on upper ribs and thumbs overlying the scapulae;

2. Move one hand anteriorly and the other hand posteriorly to induce fascial rotation and repeat for the other direction to identify rotational restriction and laxity;

3. Indirect: Rotate the cervicothoracic fascia to its position of laxity and follow any tissue release until completed;

4. Direct: Rotate the cervicothoracic fascia into its restriction and apply steady force until tissue give is completed;

5. Retest cervicothoracic rotation.

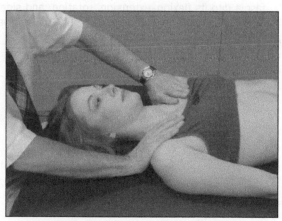

Cervicothoracic myofascial release

CERVICOTHORACIC MYOFASCIAL RELEASE—SEATED

INDICATIONS: Thoracic paraspinal tension or restricted cervicothoracic fascia related to neck pain, headache, back pain, chest wall pain, edema, shortness of breath, and other problems.

RELATIVE CONTRAINDICATIONS: Acute rib, sternum, or thoracic fracture.

TECHNIQUE (seated or supine):

1. Place one hand across the sternal angle and the other hand across the vertebra with the most tension;

2. Indirect: Gently compress the hands together and follow any fascial give to its position of laxity, maintaining fascial laxity and following any tissue release until completed;

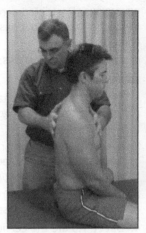

Seated cervicothoracic myofascial release

3. Direct: Gently move the cervicothoracic fascia into its flexion–extension, rotation, and sidebending restrictions and apply steady force until tissue give is completed;

4. Retest cervicothoracic motion.

THORACIC OUTLET DIRECT MYOFASCIAL RELEASE

INDICATIONS: Tension or restriction associated with neck pain, back pain, thoracic outlet syndrome, or other problems.

RELATIVE CONTRAINDICATIONS: Acute fracture, sprain, or dislocation; joint inflammation.

TECHNIQUE (supine, lateral):

1. For scalene tension, use one hand to exert inferior and lateral traction with external rotation on the arm and your other hand to move the head into its restriction in rotation and sidebending away from the side of tension, applying steady stretch until tissue give is completed;

2. For lower trapezius or triceps tension, use one hand to stabilize the head and your other hand to move the arm into its traction and rotation restrictions, applying steady stretch until tissue give is completed;

3. For pectoralis tension, use one or both hands to move the arm into its abduction and extension barriers, applying steady stretch until tissue give is completed;

4. Retest for tension or restriction.

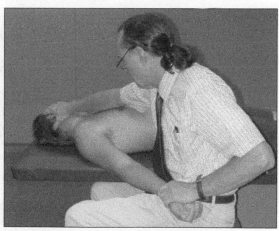

Scalene myofascial release

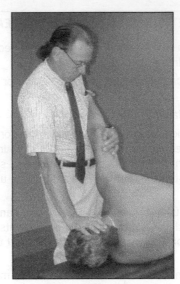

**Lower trapezius/
triceps myofascial release**

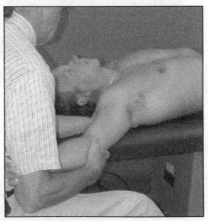

Pectoralis myofascial release

THORACIC MYOFASCIAL RELEASE

INDICATIONS: Restricted thoracic rotation related to back pain, chest wall pain, rib restriction, shoulder pain, and other problems.

RELATIVE CONTRAINDICATIONS: Acute thoracic fracture.

TECHNIQUE (supine):

1. Sitting at the head of the table, place your fingertips on the transverse processes of the restricted segment;

2. Indirect: Use your fingertips to gently move the segment to the position of rotation, sidebending, and flexion–extension laxity and follow any tissue release until completed;

3. Direct: Slowly move the segment into the rotation, sidebending, and flexion–extension restrictions and apply steady force until tissue give is completed;

4. Retest thoracic rotation.

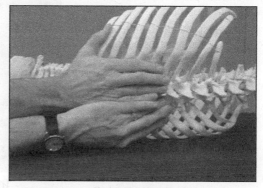

Hand placement

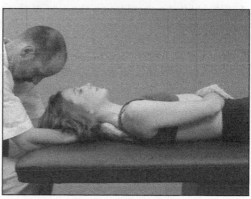

T4 myofascial release

THORACIC EXTENSION-FACILITATED POSITIONAL RELEASE[1]

INDICATIONS: Thoracic extension somatic dysfunction associated with back pain, chest wall pain, and other problems.

RELATIVE CONTRAINDICATIONS: Acute fracture, shoulder dislocation.

TECHNIQUE (prone):

1. Place a pillow under the upper chest to decrease thoracic kyphosis if desired;

2. Have the patient turn the head toward the side of thoracic rotation;

3. Stand on the opposite side of thoracic rotation and palpate the paraspinal tension;

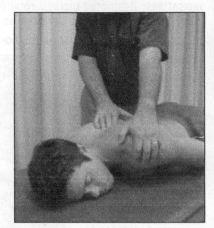

Thoracic extension facilitated positional release

4. Slowly lift the shoulder on the side of thoracic rotation toward the paraspinal tension, adding compression or torsion until tension decreases;

5. Hold this position for 3–5 seconds until tension release is completed and slowly return the shoulder to the table;

6. Remove the pillow and retest thoracic rotation.

THORACIC FLEXION-FACILITATED POSITIONAL RELEASE[1]

INDICATIONS: Thoracic flexion somatic dysfunction associated with back pain, chest wall pain, and other problems.

RELATIVE CONTRAINDICATIONS: Acute fracture.

TECHNIQUE (seated):

1. Standing behind the patient, reach over the shoulder on the side of thoracic rotation and across the upper chest to hold the top of the other shoulder;

2. Palpate the paraspinal tension and ask the patient to sit up straight to reduce thoracic kyphosis;

3. Slowly flex the trunk until motion is felt at the restricted segment;

4. Rotate the shoulders toward the side of thoracic rotation until tension decreases and add compressive force through your axilla causing sidebending at the level being monitored;

5. Hold this position for 3–5 seconds until tension release is completed and slowly return the trunk to neutral;

6. Retest thoracic rotation.

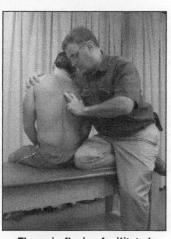

Thoracic flexion facilitated positional release for flexion, rotation and sidebending right

STERNUM LIGAMENTOUS ARTICULAR STRAIN

INDICATIONS: Sternal fascial tension or restriction associated with chest wall pain and other problems.

RELATIVE CONTRAINDICATIONS: Sternum fracture, rib fracture, and costochondral subluxation.

TECHNIQUE (supine):

1. Sit or stand at the head of the table and place the heel of your hand on the manubrium and fingertips at the xiphisternal junction;

2. Compress the sternum by pushing the manubrium posteriorly and inferiorly while pulling your fingertips posteriorly and superiorly;

3. Move the sternal fascia into its sidebending and rotation laxity;

4. Maintain sternal compression and fascial laxity, following any tissue release until completed;

5. Retest for fascial tension or restriction.

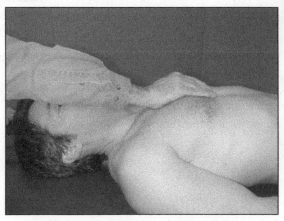

Sternum ligamentous articular strain

THORACIC PERCUSSION VIBRATOR

INDICATIONS: Thoracic somatic dysfunction associated with back pain, chest wall pain, anxiety, or other problems.

RELATIVE CONTRAINDICATIONS: Acute thoracic or rib fracture, acute shoulder sprain or surgery, shoulder inflammation, pacemaker, defibrillator, and thoracic cancer.

TECHNIQUE (lateral):

1. With the patient lying on the nonrestricted side with knees and hips flexed, place your monitoring hand over the shoulder;

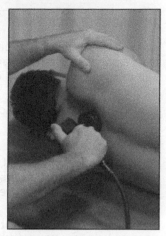
Thoracic percussion vibrator

2. Place the vibrating percussion pad lightly on the involved thoracic spinous processes perpendicular to the surface, avoiding pad bouncing;

3. Alter pad speed, pressure, and angle until vibrations are palpated as strong by the monitoring hand;

4. Maintain contact until the force and rhythm of vibration returns to that of normal tissue;

5. Alternative technique:
   a) Allow the monitoring hand to be pulled toward the pad, resisting any other direction of hand pull;
   b) Maintain percussion until the monitoring hand is pushed away from the pad;

6. Slowly release the monitoring hand and the percussion vibrator and retest tissue texture or motion.

THORACIC-SEATED FACET RELEASE

INDICATIONS: Restricted thoracic movement associated with back pain, chest wall pain, shoulder pain, and other problems.

RELATIVE CONTRAINDICATIONS: Acute thoracic fracture.

TECHNIQUE:

1. Sit behind the patient and have him or her sit up very straight so that the shoulders are balanced over the pelvis;

2. Place your forearm in front of the shoulder and pull the patient back against your abdomen;

3. Place a knuckle or finger on the inferior facet of the locked open or closed facet group;

4. Gently compress inferiorly through the shoulder while keeping the shoulders balanced over the pelvis. Repeat for the other shoulder to determine the side of facet restriction;

5. Test the side of facet restriction for the position of greatest restriction by gentle compression and recoil on the shoulder to close and open the locked facet;

6. Hold the patient in the position of greatest restriction and gently induce a small amount of additional compression or traction through the shoulder to induce glide of the facet, thereby releasing the restriction;

7. Retest thoracic motion.

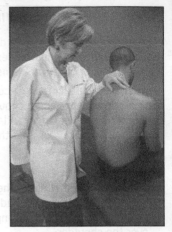

Initial positioning

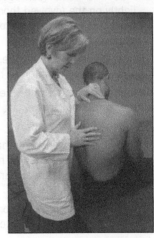

Compression of left facet

UPPER THORACIC-SEATED FACET RELEASE

INDICATIONS: Restricted upper thoracic movement associated with back pain, chest wall pain, shoulder pain, neck pain, headache, and other problems.

RELATIVE CONTRAINDICATIONS: Acute cervical or thoracic fracture, acute cervical sprain, and restricted or painful shoulder (alternative positioning).

TECHNIQUE:

1. Stand behind the patient and increase upper thoracic kyphosis by flexing the head and having the patient lean back into you, keeping the shoulders balanced over the pelvis;

Initial positioning

2. Place your thumb on the inferior facet of the locked open or closed facet group;

3. Place your other hand on the head and gently compress inferiorly, positioning the cervical spine to localize the compression at the facet being tested and keeping the shoulders balanced over the pelvis. Repeat for the other side to determine the side of facet restriction;

4. Test the side of facet restriction for the position of greatest restriction by gentle compression and recoil on the head to close and open the locked facet;

5. Hold the patient in the position of greatest restriction and gently induce a small amount of additional compression or traction through the head to induce glide of the facet, thereby releasing the restriction. Alternative positioning uses opposite arm to induce compression and recoil;

6. Retest upper thoracic motion.

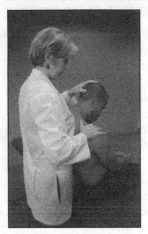

Compression for right T2

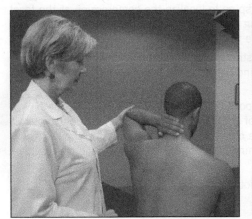
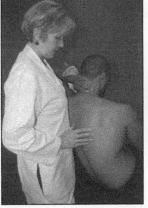

Alternative upper thoracic positioning

THORACIC MUSCLE ENERGY/THRUST—SEATED

INDICATIONS: Restricted thoracic rotation related to back pain, chest wall pain, shoulder pain, or other problems.

RELATIVE CONTRAINDICATIONS: Joint inflammation, acute sprain, acute fracture, vertebral cancer, and vertebral fusion (thrust only).

TECHNIQUE:

1. Standing behind the seated patient, place your thenar eminence or thumb on the posterior transverse process(es);

2. Reach across the upper chest with your other hand and arm to control the patient's shoulders and trunk. For T1–4 restrictions hold the top of the head to induce cervical and upper thoracic motion;

3. Move the trunk or head into the rotation, sidebending, and flexion–extension restrictive barriers until you feel movement at the restricted segment(s);

4. Ask the patient to straighten out the trunk or head for 3–5 seconds against your equal resistance;

5. Allow full relaxation and slowly move the trunk or head to new restrictive barriers as you push anteriorly into the posterior transverse process(es);

6. Repeat this isometric contraction and stretch 3–5 times or until thoracic mobility returns;

7. For T5–12, a thrust can be added if needed by a short and quick anterior push into the posterior transverse process(es) as you simultaneously move the trunk into its barriers;

8. Retest thoracic rotation. If successful, consider prescribing THORACIC FLEXION/EXTENSION STRETCH.

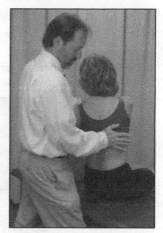

Muscle energy for T7 flexed, rotated and sidebent right

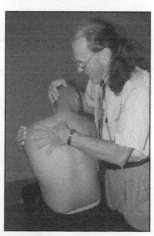

Muscle energy for T2 extended, rotated and sidebent left

THORACIC FLEXION/EXTENSION STRETCH[2]

1. Kneel with your arms straight and hands shoulder width apart;
2. Arch your back slowly upward while tucking the head and tailbone down;
3. Take a few deep breaths and stretch for 5–10 seconds;

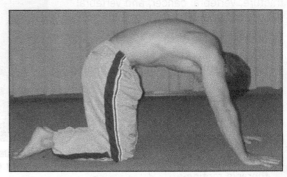

Thoracic flexion stretch

4. Arch your back slowly downward while curling the head and tailbone upward;
5. Take a few deep breaths and stretch for 5–10 seconds;
6. Repeat 3–5 times;
7. Do these stretches 1–4 times a day.

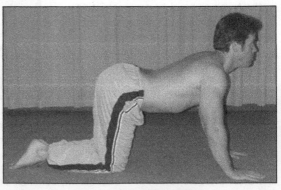

Thoracic extension stretch

THORACIC/RIB ARTICULATORY—SUPINE

INDICATIONS: Restricted thoracic rotation or rib motion related to back pain, chest wall pain, shoulder pain, or other problems.

RELATIVE CONTRAINDICATIONS: Joint inflammation, joint hypermobility, acute sprain, acute fracture, and vertebral cancer.

TECHNIQUE (supine):

Supine thoracic articulatory

1. Stand at the head of the patient whose hands are clasped behind the head;
2. Reach through the patients arms and hold the back of the rib cage;
3. Lift the upper back and place your bent knee under the restricted area;
4. Use your arms and body to slowly roll the patient backward over your knee while lifting the rib cage to mobilize the restricted joints;
5. Repeat for other restricted areas;
6. Retest thoracic rotation.

THORACIC THRUST—PRONE

INDICATIONS: Restricted thoracic rotation related to back pain, chest wall pain, shoulder pain, or other problems.

RELATIVE CONTRAINDICATIONS: Joint inflammation, joint hypermobility, acute sprain, acute fracture, vertebral cancer, and vertebral fusion.

TECHNIQUE:

1. Stand on the side of thoracic rotation and place your hypothenar eminence on the posterior transverse process;
2. Place the thenar eminence of your other hand on the opposite transverse process of the segment above or below the one being treated;
3. Ask the patient to take a deep breath and follow exhalation with gentle anterior pressure from both hands;
4. At the end of exhalation, apply a short quick thrust in an anterior direction with both hands;
5. Retest thoracic rotation.

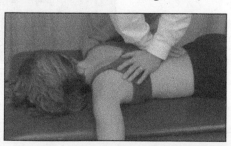

Prone thrust for T8 rotated right

THORACIC/RIB THRUST—SUPINE

INDICATIONS: Restricted thoracic rotation or rib motion related to back pain, chest wall pain, shoulder pain, or other problems.

RELATIVE CONTRAINDICATIONS: Joint inflammation, joint hypermobility, acute sprain, acute fracture, costochondral subluxation, vertebral cancer, vertebral fusion, and severe osteoporosis.

TECHNIQUE:

1. Stand on the opposite side of thoracic rotation or rib restriction;

2. Cross the patient's arms with the elbows together and the arm on the side of thoracic rotation on top;

3. Reach your caudad arm across the patient and place the thenar eminence behind the posterior transverse process or rib angle;

4. Lean your epigastric area into the patient's crossed elbows;

5. Use your other hand to lift the patient's head and trunk until pressure from leaning on the elbows is felt by your thenar eminence;

6. Ask the patient to take a deep breath, lean into the elbows during exhalation, and at maximum exhalation quickly drop your abdomen onto the elbows to mobilize the joint;

7. Retest thoracic or rib motion. If successful, consider prescribing THORACIC SELF-MOBILIZATION—SUPINE.

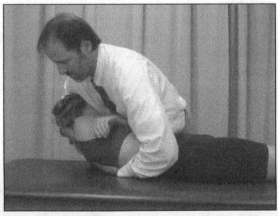

Supine thrust for T8 rotated right

THORACIC/RIB SELF-MOBILIZATION—SUPINE[2]

1. Lie on your back with knees bent and fingers locked behind the head;
2. Push your elbows together. For ribs, roll the arms to one side;
3. Use your arms to pull the head forward while simultaneously lifting the pelvis until a single vertebra or rib touches the floor;
4. Rock the pelvis up and down to roll a vertebra over the floor until a mobilization is felt;
5. Repeat for other vertebrae or ribs if needed;
6. Do this mobilization up to twice a day.

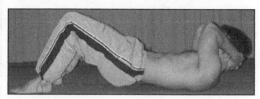

Thoracic self-mobilization—supine

THORACIC/RIB THRUST—SEATED

INDICATIONS: Restricted thoracic rotation or rib mobility related to back pain, chest wall pain, shoulder pain, or other problems.

RELATIVE CONTRAINDICATIONS: Joint inflammation, joint hypermobility, acute sprain, acute fracture, vertebral cancer, and vertebral fusion.

TECHNIQUE:

1. Stand behind the patient whose hands are clasped behind the head;
2. Place your epigastric area behind the posterior transverse process or rib angle;

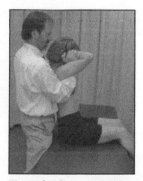

Thoracic/rib seated thrust

3. Reach under the patient's arms and hold the forearms;
4. Ask the patient to take a deep breath and during exhalation pull the elbows together, extend the trunk, and push your abdomen into the posterior transverse process or rib;
5. At maximal exhalation, apply a short quick thrust with your abdomen into the posterior transverse process or rib angle;
6. Retest thoracic rotation or rib motion. If successful, consider prescribing THORACIC SELF-MOBILIZATION—KNEELING or THORACIC SELF-MOBILIZATION—STANDING.

THORACIC SELF-MOBILIZATION—KNEELING

1. Kneel with your arms straight and hands shoulder width;
2. Reach your left shoulder down toward the left hip as far as it will go;
3. Reach your right shoulder down toward the right hip as far as it will go;
4. Repeat 3–5 times;
5. Do this mobilization up to twice a day.

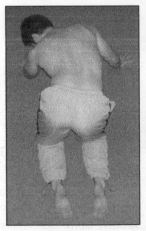

Thoracic self-mobilization—kneeling

THORACIC SELF-MOBILIZATION—STANDING[3]

1. Stand with arms hanging by your side;

2. Swing your arms to one side, allowing the back to follow as far as it will go;

3. Swing your arms to the other side, allowing the back to follow as far as it will go;

4. Repeat 3–5 times;

5. Clasp the hands behind your head;

6. Swing your arms to one side, allowing the head and upper back to follow as far as they will go;

7. Swing your arms to the other side, allowing the head and upper back to follow as far as they will go;

8. Repeat 3–5 times;

9. Do these mobilizations up to twice a day.

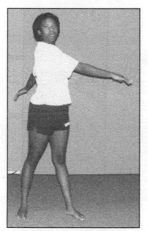

Lower thoracic self-mobilization

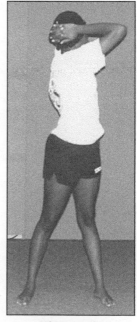

Mid-thoracic self-mobilization

REFERENCES

1. Adapted from Schiowitz S, DiGiovanna EL, Dowling DJ. Facilitated positional release [Chapter 64]. In: Ward RC, ed. *Foundations for Osteopathic Medicine*. 2nd ed. Philadelphia, PA: Lippincott Williams & Wilkins; 2003.
2. Adapted from Kirk CE. *Biodynamics of Self-Administered Manipulation*. *1977 AAO Yearbook*. Colorado Springs, CO: American Academy of Osteopathy, 1979.
3. Adapted from Steiner CS. Tennis elbow. *J Am Osteopath Assoc* 1976;75(6):575–581.

8 Rib Diagnosis and Treatment

Diagnosis of Rib Somatic Dysfunction
1. Rib angle palpation *p. 168*
2. Rib tender points *p. 169*
3. Rib motion testing *p. 170*
4. Thoracic/rib diagnosis using inherent motion *p. 171*
5. Rib somatic dysfunction (Table 8-1) *p. 172*

Treatment of Rib Somatic Dysfunction
1. OMT
   Rib 1 counterstrain *p. 173*
   Rib 1 seated facet release *p. 174*
   Rib 1 articulatory *p. 176*
   Rib 1 muscle energy/thrust—supine *p. 177*
   Rib 1 thrust—prone *p. 178*
   Rib 1 thrust—seated *p. 178*
   Posterior rib 2–10 counterstrain *p. 179*
   Anterior rib 1–2 counterstrain *p. 180*
   Anterior rib 3–10 counterstrain *p. 181*
   Rib myofascial release *p. 182*
   Rib myofascial release using shoulder *p. 183*
   Focal inhibition facilitated oscillatory release *p. 184*
   Rib percussion vibrator *p. 185*
   Rib seated facet release *p. 186*
   Rib subluxation muscle energy *p. 187*
   Rib inhalation muscle energy *p. 188*
   Rib exhalation muscle energy *p. 189*
   Rib 11–12 muscle energy *p. 192*
   Rib 11–12 thrust *p. 194*
2. Exercises
   Rib 1 self-mobilization *p. 179*
   Posterior rib position of ease *p. 180*
   Anterior rib position of ease *p. 181*
   Pectoralis stretch *p. 191*
   Latissimus stretch *p. 191*

167

Diagnosis

RIB ANGLE PALPATION

1. Flex and adduct one arm to move the scapula away from the posterior chest wall;

2. Palpate for symmetry and tenderness of the rib angles which become progressively lateral in the lower rib cage;

3. The following findings indicate the listed somatic dysfunctions:

   a) Prominent rib angle = posterior rib subluxation;
   b) Depressed rib angle = anterior rib subluxation;
   c) Tender rib angle = elevated rib tender point, rib subluxation, or key rib.

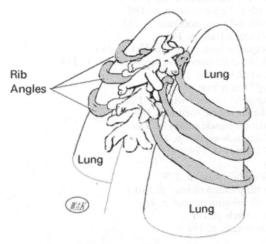

**A rib angle is the posterior prominence
(Drawing by William A. Kuchera, DO, FAAO)**

RIB TENDER POINTS

1. Palpate for posterior (elevated) rib tender points at the following locations:

   a) **Posterior rib 1**—lateral shaft anterior to trapezius muscle;

   b) **Posterior ribs 2–7**—rib angles with scapula rotated away by flexing and adducting arm;

   c) **Posterior ribs 8–10**—rib angles which are more lateral with each lower rib.

2. Palpate for anterior (depressed) rib tender points at the following locations:

   a) **Anterior rib 1**—inferior to medial clavicle, lateral to sternum;

   b) **Anterior rib 2**—rib shaft in mid-clavicular line;

   c) **Anterior ribs 3–10**—rib shaft in anterior axillary line or mid-axillary line.

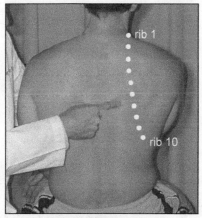

**Posterior rib tender points
(right PT8 shown)**

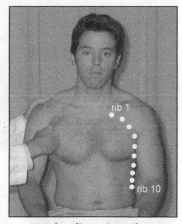

**Anterior rib tender points
(pectoralis minor palpation shown)**

RIB MOTION TESTING

1. Let your fingers rest gently on the shafts of the ribs being assessed:
   a) Rib 1—first fingers at the base of the lateral neck just anterior to the trapezius muscle;
   b) Ribs 2–5—fingers on anteromedial shafts along the sternum;
   c) Ribs 6–10—fingers on the lateral shafts in the mid-axillary line;
   d) Ribs 11–12—first and second fingers on shafts posteriorly;
2. Ask the patient to breathe deeply in and out and passively follow rib motion (see Fig. p.171);
3. Restricted rib exhalation—inhalation somatic dysfunction;
4. Restricted rib inhalation—exhalation somatic dysfunction.

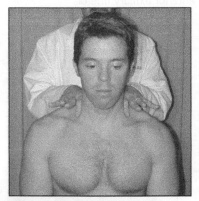

Rib 1

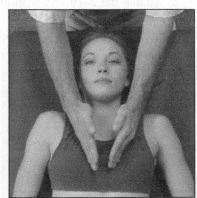

Ribs 2–5

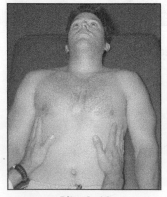

Ribs 6–10

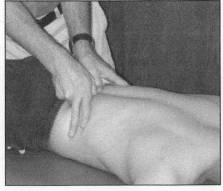

Ribs 11–12

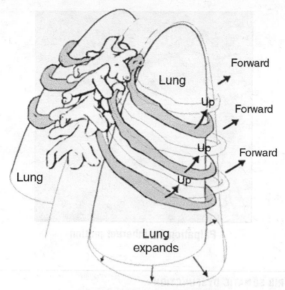

Rib motion with inhalation
(Drawing by William A. Kuchera, DO, FAAO)

THORACIC/RIB DIAGNOSIS USING INHERENT MOTION*

1. With the patient supine, place your hands gently over the lower ribs;

2. Palpate inherent flexion (rib inhalation) and extension (rib exhalation) to identify restricted motion;

   a) Restricted bilateral flexion indicates restricted thoracic extension;
   b) Restricted unilateral flexion indicates rib exhalation ease or thoracic rotation ease to the opposite side;
   c) Restricted bilateral extension indicates restricted thoracic flexion;
   d) Restricted unilateral extension indicates rib inhalation ease or thoracic rotation ease to the same side;

3. If related to the patient problem, treat the restriction with myofascial release, balanced membranous tension, or other techniques.

---

*The term inherent motion refers to a palpable cyclic pressure fluctuation variably referred to as cranial rhythmic impulse, craniosacral motion, entrainment, primary respiratory mechanism, pulse pressure fluctuation, and Traube–Hering–Mayer wave.

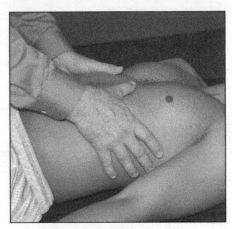

Palpation for inherent motion

Table 8-1	RIB SOMATIC DYSFUNCTION	
Somatic Dysfunction	**Diagnostic Finding**	**Key Rib[a]**
Posterior tender point	Tenderness at rib angle Tenderness on rib shaft	Most tender rib
Anterior tender point	At anterior or mid-axillary line	Most tender rib
Posterior subluxation	Prominent rib angle	
Anterior subluxation	Anterior rib angle	
Inhalation somatic dysfunction[b]	Restricted exhalation	Inferior rib
Exhalation somatic dysfunction[b]	Restricted inhalation	Superior rib

[a]The key rib is the rib in a group somatic dysfunction which can be treated first to allow resolution of associated rib somatic dysfunctions.

[b]For rib 1, inhalation somatic dysfunction is termed an elevated first rib and exhalation somatic dysfunction is termed a depressed first rib.

Treatment

RIB 1 COUNTERSTRAIN

INDICATIONS: Posterior (elevated) rib 1 tender point associated with shoulder pain, neck pain, headache, thoracic outlet syndrome, and other problems.

RELATIVE CONTRAINDICATIONS: Acute cervical fracture.

TECHNIQUE (seated):

1. Locate the tender point on the shaft of the first rib at the lower neck just anterior to the upper trapezius muscle, labeling it 10/10;

2. Place your foot on the table on the side of the tender point and drape the patient's arm over your thigh;

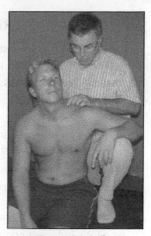

Elevated left first rib counterstrain

3. Make the patient lean onto your thigh, sidebend the head toward the tender point, and retest for tenderness;

4. Fine tune this position with slight cervical extension and rotation until tenderness is minimized to 0/10 if possible but at most to 3/10;

5. Hold the position of maximum relief for 120 seconds, maintaining finger contact to monitor for tissue texture changes but reducing pressure;

6. Slowly and passively return to neutral and retest for tenderness with the same pressure as initial labeling.

RIB 1 SEATED FACET RELEASE

INDICATIONS: Restricted first rib associated with back pain, chest wall pain, shoulder pain, neck pain, headache, and other problems.

RELATIVE CONTRAINDICATIONS: Acute cervical or thoracic fracture, acute cervical sprain.

TECHNIQUE:

1. Stand behind the patient and increase upper thoracic kyphosis by flexing the head and having the patient lean back onto you;

2. Place your thumb at the costotransverse facet of the first rib;

3. Place your other hand on the head and gently compress inferiorly while positioning the cervical spine to test each first rib;

4. Test the side of rib restriction for the position of greatest restriction by gently inducing compression on the head and allowing recoil to close and open the locked facet;

5. Hold the patient in the position of greatest restriction and gently induce a small amount of additional compression or traction through the head to induce glide of the facet, thereby releasing the restriction. Alternative positioning uses opposite arm to induce compression and recoil (see UPPER THORACIC SEATED FACET RELEASE,) p. 157

6. Retest first rib motion.

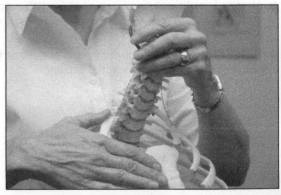

Thumb position

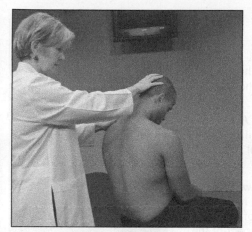

Initial positioning

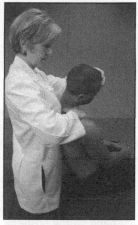

Testing with compression

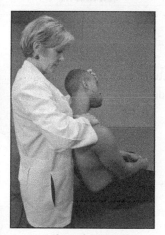

Testing with recoil

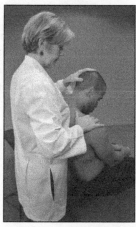

Compression of right first rib

RIB 1 ARTICULATORY

INDICATIONS: Restricted rib 1 exhalation associated with neck pain, headache, thoracic outlet syndrome, shoulder pain, or other problems.

RELATIVE CONTRAINDICATIONS: Acute sprain or fracture, rib 1 hypermobility, dizziness or nausea with cervical rotation.

TECHNIQUE (seated):

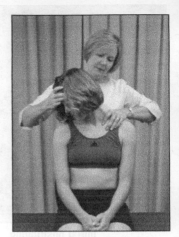

Articulatory for elevated left first rib

1. Hold the patient's head with one hand and place the first metacarpal–phalangeal (MCP) joint of your other hand on the posterior aspect of the elevated first rib;

2. Push the rib inferomedially while you slowly move the head into sidebending away from the rib, extension, and sidebending toward the rib, and flexion in one smooth motion;

3. Repeat 3–5 times or until rib mobility returns;

4. Retest rib 1 motion. If successful, consider prescribing RIB 1 SELF-MOBILIZATION.

RIB 1 MUSCLE ENERGY/THRUST—SUPINE

INDICATIONS: Restricted first rib exhalation associated with neck pain, headache, thoracic outlet syndrome, shoulder pain, or other problems.

RELATIVE CONTRAINDICATIONS: Acute cervical sprain or fracture, undiagnosed cervical radiculopathy, vertebral cancer, rib 1 hypermobility (thrust only).

TECHNIQUE:

1. Hold the occiput in your palms and place your first metacarpal–phalangeal (MCP) joint at the posterolateral aspect of the elevated first rib with that arm pointing toward the opposite axilla;

2. Push the rib in an anteromedial and inferior direction as you sidebend the head around your MCP joint and rotate the head to the opposite side;

3. Ask the patient to straighten the head for 3–5 seconds against your equal resistance;

4. Repeat this isometric contraction and relaxation 3–5 times or until rib mobilization occurs;

5. If needed, apply a short and quick thrust into the rib toward the opposite axilla;

6. Retest rib 1 motion. If successful, consider prescribing RIB 1 SELF-MOBILIZATION.

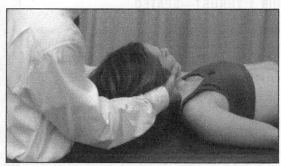

Supine muscle energy/thrust for elevated right first rib

RIB 1 THRUST—PRONE

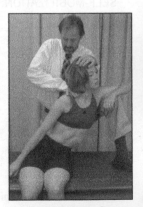

INDICATIONS: Restricted first rib exhalation associated with neck pain, headache, thoracic outlet syndrome, shoulder pain, or other problems.

RELATIVE CONTRAINDICATIONS: Acute cervical sprain or fracture, rib 1 hypermobility, undiagnosed cervical radiculopathy, vertebral cancer.

TECHNIQUE:

1. Stand at the head of the prone patient whose chin is on the table;

Prone thrust for elevated right first rib

2. Reach across the head and place your thenar or hypothenar eminence on the posterior aspect of the elevated first rib, pushing toward the anterior superior iliac spine (ASIS) on the same side;

3. Reach under your arm with the other hand and slowly roll the head into a sidebending restrictive barrier away from the elevated rib;

4. Apply a short quick thrust onto the rib toward the ipsilateral ASIS;

5. Retest first rib motion. If successful, consider prescribing RIB 1 SELF-MOBILIZATION.

RIB 1 THRUST—SEATED

INDICATIONS: Restricted first rib exhalation associated with neck pain, headache, thoracic outlet syndrome, shoulder pain, or other problems.

RELATIVE CONTRAINDICATIONS: Acute sprain or fracture, rib 1 hypermobility, undiagnosed cervical radiculopathy, vertebral cancer.

TECHNIQUE:

1. Place your first metacarpal–phalangeal joint on the posterolateral aspect of the elevated first rib, hold the patient's head with your other hand, and lean the patient away from the elevated rib by draping his or her arm over your thigh with your foot on the table;

Seated thrust for elevated right first rib

2. Push the rib in an anteromedial and inferior direction, sidebend the head toward the elevated rib, lean the patient farther over your thigh, and apply a short quick thrust into the rib toward the opposite axilla;

3. Retest rib 1 motion. If successful, consider prescribing RIB 1 SELF-MOBILIZATION.

RIB 1 SELF-MOBILIZATION

1. Sit with one hand firmly holding the top of the other shoulder at the base of the neck on the side of the restricted rib;

2. Slowly move your head in a circle, bending toward the hand, forward, away from the hand, backward, and toward the hand again. Stop if dizziness, nausea, or blurred vision occurs;

3. Repeat until first rib movement occurs;

4. Do this mobilization up to twice a day.

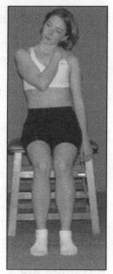

Left first rib self-mobilization

POSTERIOR RIB 2–10 COUNTERSTRAIN

INDICATIONS: Posterior rib tender point associated with back pain, chest wall pain, and other problems.

RELATIVE CONTRAINDICATIONS: Acute thoracic or rib sprain or fracture.

TECHNIQUE (seated):

1. Locate the tender point on the posterior rib angle, labeling it 10/10;

2. Place your foot on the table to the side of the tender point and drape the patient's arm over your thigh;

3. Make the patient lean onto your thigh, and retest for tenderness;

4. Fine tune this position with more sidebending and slight trunk rotation until tenderness is minimized to 0/10 if possible but at the most to 3/10;

5. Hold the position of maximum relief for 120 seconds, maintaining finger contact to monitor for tissue texture changes but reducing pressure;

6. Slowly and passively return to neutral and retest for tenderness with the same pressure as initial labeling. If successful, consider prescribing POSTERIOR RIB POSITION OF EASE.

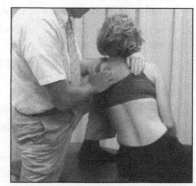

Posterior left third rib counterstrain

POSTERIOR RIB POSITION OF EASE

1. Sit with your arm on the side of back pain resting on a table or counter;
2. Lean toward the table until pain is reduced;
3. If comfortable, take a few deep breaths and rest in this position for 2–5 minutes;
4. Slowly sit back up and let the arm drop to your side;
5. Repeat 2–4 times a day or as needed for pain relief.

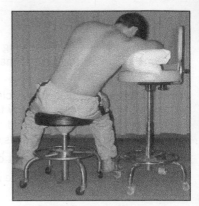

Position of ease for right posterior rib

ANTERIOR RIB 1–2 COUNTERSTRAIN

INDICATIONS: Anterior rib 1 or 2 tender point associated with chest wall pain, neck pain, and other problems.

RELATIVE CONTRAINDICATIONS: Acute cervical or rib fracture or dislocation.

TECHNIQUE (supine):

1. Locate the tender point inferior to the clavicle and just lateral to the sternum (rib 1) or in the mid-clavicular line (rib 2), labeling it 10/10;

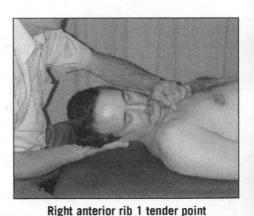

Right anterior rib 1 tender point and treatment position

2. Flex the head, rotate, and sidebend it toward the tender point, and retest for tenderness;
3. Fine tune this position with slight changes in flexion, sidebending, and rotation until tenderness is minimized to 0/10 if possible but at the most to 3/10;
4. Hold the position of maximum relief for 120 seconds, maintaining finger contact to monitor for tissue texture changes but reducing pressure;
5. Slowly and passively return to neutral and retest for tenderness with the same pressure as initial labeling.

ANTERIOR RIB 3–10 COUNTERSTRAIN

INDICATIONS: Anterior rib tender point associated with chest wall pain and other problems.

RELATIVE CONTRAINDICATIONS: Acute thoracic or rib sprain or fracture.

TECHNIQUE (seated):

1. Locate the anterior rib tender point, labeling 10/10;

2. Place your foot on the table to the opposite side of the tender point and drape the patient's arm over your thigh;

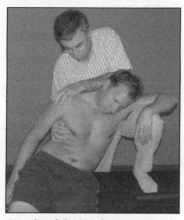

Anterior right 6th rib counterstrain

3. Lean the patient onto your thigh and retest for tenderness;

4. Fine tune this position with more sidebending and slight trunk rotation until tenderness is minimized to 0/10 if possible but at the most to 3/10;

5. Hold the position of maximum relief for 120 seconds, maintaining finger contact to monitor for tissue texture changes but reducing pressure;

6. Slowly and passively return to neutral and retest for tenderness with the same pressure as initial labeling. If successful, consider prescribing ANTERIOR RIB POSITION OF EASE.

ANTERIOR RIB POSITION OF EASE

1. Sit with your arm on the pain free side resting on a table or counter;

2. Lean toward the table until pain is reduced;

3. If comfortable, rest in this position for 2–5 minutes;

4. Slowly sit back up and let the arm fall to your side;

5. Repeat 2–4 times a day or as needed for pain relief.

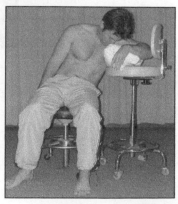

Position of ease for right anterior rib

RIB MYOFASCIAL RELEASE

INDICATIONS: Rib somatic dysfunction related to back pain, chest wall pain, and other problems.

RELATIVE CONTRAINDICATIONS: Acute rib fracture.

TECHNIQUE (seated or supine):

1. Hold the involved rib angle with two fingers of one hand and the anterior rib with two fingers of your other hand, placing your thumbs along the lateral rib;

2. Apply gentle anterior–posterior compression between your hands until any tissue give is completed;

3. Apply gentle lateral traction to the entire rib and follow any tissue release until completed;

4. Slowly release the rib and retest rib motion.

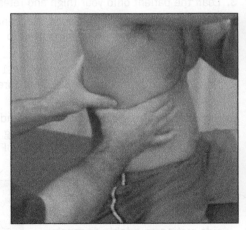

Rib myofascial release

RIB MYOFASCIAL RELEASE USING SHOULDER

INDICATIONS: Rib restriction or tender point related to back pain, chest wall pain, and other problems.

RELATIVE CONTRAINDICATIONS: Acute rib fracture, acute shoulder sprain, shoulder joint inflammation.

TECHNIQUE (supine):

1. Sitting at the head of the table, reach behind the shoulder with one hand and pull the involved rib angle superiorly;

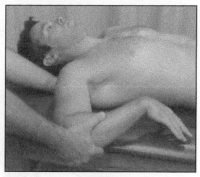
Abduction

2. Grasp the proximal forearm and slowly abduct the arm while maintaining shoulder internal rotation and superior pull on the rib, holding steady force at any restriction until tissue give is completed (see LATISSIMUS DORSI MUSCLE, *p. 184*);

3. Slowly externally rotate the arm and move it into additional abduction while maintaining superior pull on the rib, holding steady force at any restriction until tissue give is completed;

4. Slowly adduct the arm while maintaining arm external rotation and superior pull on the rib, holding steady force at any restriction until tissue give is completed and placing the arm at the patient's side;

5. Maintaining superior pull on the rib, move your other hand from the forearm to the shoulder and repetitively compress the shoulder toward the rib for 10 to 20 seconds or until rib movement occurs;

6. Slowly return the arm to the table and retest rib motion.

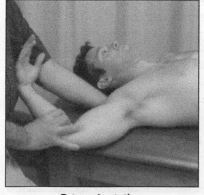
External rotation

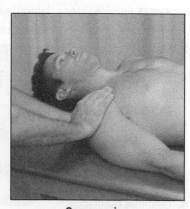
Compression

LATISSIMUS DORSI MUSCLE

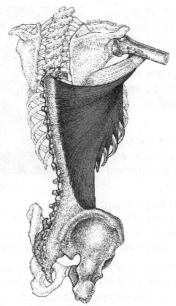

Attachments to ribs 8–12

FOCAL INHIBITION FACILITATED OSCILLATORY RELEASE

INDICATIONS: Tissue tension or tenderness associated with pain, restricted mobility, or other problems.

RELATIVE CONTRAINDICATIONS: Acute fracture, significant patient guarding.

TECHNIQUE (supine, prone, lateral, seated):

1. Place one or two fingertips on the target tissue;

2. Use your other hand to apply positional stretch by moving the body or skin away from the target tissue;

3. Initiate oscillatory force through the fingertips into the target tissue by rhythmically moving your forearm;

4. Continue oscillation until tension is reduced.

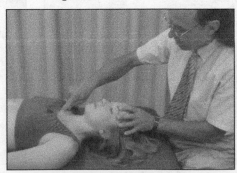

Focal inhibition for intercostal muscle

RIB PERCUSSION VIBRATOR

INDICATIONS: Rib somatic dysfunction associated with chest wall pain, back pain, shortness of breath, cough, and other problems.

CONTRAINDICATIONS: Acute rib fracture or costochondral separation, pacemaker, defibrillator, rib cancer, pregnancy.

TECHNIQUE (supine):

1. Place your monitoring hand on the left mid-axillary line at the level of rib somatic dysfunction;
2. Place the vibrating percussion pad lightly on a depression in the right mid-axillary line at the level of rib somatic dysfunction;
3. Alter pad speed, pressure, and angle until vibrations are palpated as strong by the monitoring hand;
4. Maintain contact until the force and rhythm of vibration returns to that of a normal tissue;
5. Alternative technique:
   a) Allow the monitoring hand to be pulled toward the pad, resisting any other direction of hand pull;
   b) Maintain percussion until the monitoring hand is pushed away from the pad;
6. Slowly release the monitoring hand and the percussion vibrator and retest for rib somatic dysfunction.

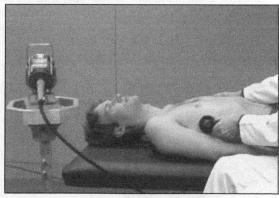

Rib 6 percussion vibrator

RIB SEATED FACET RELEASE

INDICATIONS: Restricted rib motion associated with back pain, chest wall pain, shoulder pain, and other problems.

RELATIVE CONTRAINDICATIONS: Acute thoracic or rib fracture.

TECHNIQUE:

1. Stand behind the patient and have him or her sit up very straight so that the shoulders are balanced over the pelvis;

2. Place a thumb at the costotransverse articulation;

3. Place your forearm anterior to the ipsilateral shoulder and gently compress posteriorly to firmly support the patient against your torso;

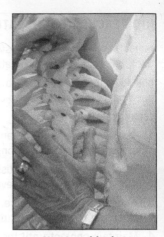
Hand positioning

4. Test for the position of greatest restriction by gentle compression and recoil through the shoulder to close and open the locked facet while keeping the patient firmly held against your torso;

5. Hold the patient in the position of greatest restriction and gently induce a small amount of additional compression or traction through the shoulder to induce glide of the costotransverse facet, thereby releasing the restriction. Translation of your body with the patient firmly pinned against you may aid in inducing compression or traction. Alternative positioning uses the arm to induce compression and recoil [see UPPER THORACIC SEATED FACET RELEASE, p. 157.]

6. Retest rib motion.

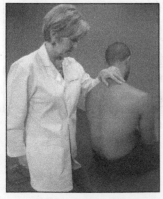
Initial positioning

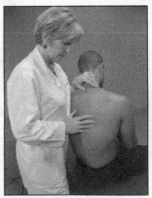
Compression of left facet

RIB SUBLUXATION MUSCLE ENERGY

INDICATIONS: Anterior or posterior rib subluxation associated with chest wall pain, back pain, shoulder pain, and other problems.

RELATIVE CONTRAINDICATIONS: Severe osteoporosis, acute rib fracture, acute costochondral subluxation, vertebral or rib cancer.

TECHNIQUE (seated):

1. Stand behind the patient and use your thenar eminence or thumb to push the involved rib as follows:
   a) Posterior subluxation—push the rib angle anteromedially;
   b) Anterior subluxation—push the costotransverse articulation posterolaterally;

2. Ask the patient to push the flexed elbow as follows for 3–5 seconds against your equal resistance:
   a) Posterior subluxation—the patient pushes the elbow medially;
   b) Anterior subluxation—the patient pushes the elbow laterally;

3. Allow full relaxation and then increase pressure on the rib until give stops;

4. Repeat this isometric contraction and stretch 3–5 times or until rib symmetry returns;

5. Retest rib angle symmetry.

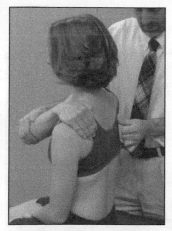

Posterior subluxation

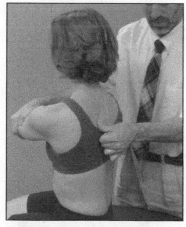

Anterior subluxation

RIB INHALATION MUSCLE ENERGY

INDICATIONS: Rib exhalation restriction associated with chest wall pain, back pain, shoulder pain, and other problems.

RELATIVE CONTRAINDICATIONS: Severe osteoporosis, acute rib fracture, acute costochondral subluxation, vertebral or rib cancer.

TECHNIQUE (supine):

1. Sit or stand at the head of the supine patient;

2. Use your palm, thumb, or fingers to push inferiorly on the shaft of the inferior rib in the group:

   a) Ribs 2–5—push inferiorly on rib shaft in the anterior axillary line. Avoid breast contact for a female patient by pushing on the medial aspect of the rib near the sternum or onto her hand placed on the rib shaft (shown below);

   b) Ribs 6–10—push inferiorly on rib shaft in the mid-axillary line;

3. Use your other hand to flex and sidebend the neck and thorax until inferior motion is felt at the inferior rib in the group;

4. Ask the patient to inhale deeply while you resist superior rib movement;

5. During exhalation push the rib more inferiorly as you flex and sidebend the neck and thorax a little farther;

6. Repeat this isometric contraction and stretch 3–5 times or until rib motion returns;

7. Retest rib motion.

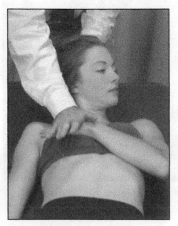

Ribs 2–5 inhalation

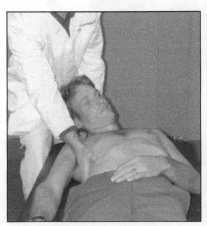

Ribs 6–10 inhalation

RIB EXHALATION MUSCLE ENERGY

INDICATIONS: Rib inhalation restriction associated with chest wall pain, back pain, shoulder pain, and other problems.

RELATIVE CONTRAINDICATIONS: Severe osteoporosis, acute rib fracture, acute costochondral subluxation, vertebral or rib cancer.

TECHNIQUE (supine):

1. Sit on the side of the rib restriction and use the fingers of one hand to pull inferiorly on the rib angle of the superior rib in the group;

2. Ask the patient to push for 3–5 seconds against your equal resistance:
   a) Rib 2—flex the head which is rotated slightly away (posterior scalene contraction);
   b) Ribs 3–5—push the elbow of the abducted arm across the chest (pectoralis minor contraction—see PECTORALIS MINOR MUSCLE, *p. 190*);
   c) Ribs 6–10—push the abducted arm down toward the side (serratus anterior contraction);

3. Allow full relaxation and then pull the rib angle inferiorly to a new barrier;

4. Repeat this isometric contraction and stretch 3–5 times or until rib motion returns;

5. Retest rib motion, if successful consider prescribing PECTORALIS STRETCH or LATISSIMUS STRETCH.

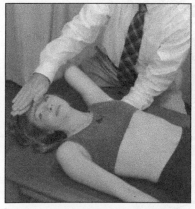

Muscle energy for rib 2 exhalation

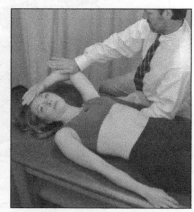

Muscle energy for ribs 3–5

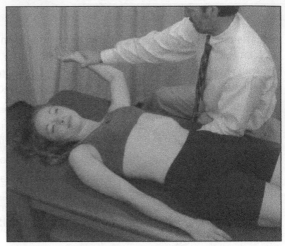

Muscle energy for ribs 6–10

PECTORALIS MINOR MUSCLE

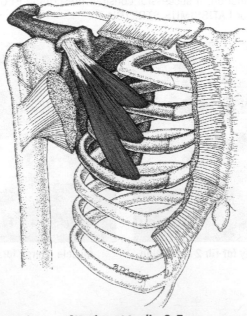

Attachment to ribs 3–5

PECTORALIS STRETCH

1. Kneel with your hands flat on the floor slightly in front of your head;
2. Squat back toward your heels as far as you can while keeping the arms straight and letting the chest drop down toward the floor;
3. Take a few deep breaths and stretch for 10–20 seconds;
4. Do this stretch 1–4 times a day.

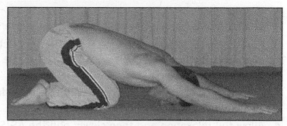

Pectoral stretch

LATISSIMUS STRETCH

1. Stand with your feet shoulder width apart;
2. Place one arm behind your head;
3. With the other hand grasp the elbow, and slowly lean your trunk away from the arm behind the head;
4. Take a few deep breaths and stretch for 10–20 seconds;
5. Repeat for the other side;
6. Do this stretch 1–4 times a day.

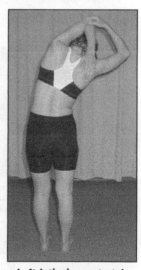

Left latissimus stretch

RIB 11–12 MUSCLE ENERGY

INDICATIONS: Rib 11 or 12 restriction associated with back pain, chest wall pain, and other problems.

RELATIVE CONTRAINDICATIONS: Acute rib fracture, vertebral or rib cancer.

TECHNIQUE (prone):

1. Stand on the opposite side of the restricted rib and place your thumb on the inferior aspect of the rib to create a fulcrum:
   a) Inhalation restriction—thumb on rib shaft;
   b) Exhalation restriction—thumb on costotransverse articulation;

2. Pull the ASIS posteriorly on the side of rib restriction to stretch the quadratus lumborum muscle until give stops (see QUADRATUS LUMBORUM MUSCLE, *p. 193*);

3. Ask the patient to push the hip toward the table for 3–5 seconds against your equal resistance;

4. Allow full relaxation and then slowly pull the ASIS posteriorly until tissue give stops;

5. Repeat this isometric contraction and stretch 3–5 times or until rib motion returns;

6. Retest rib motion.

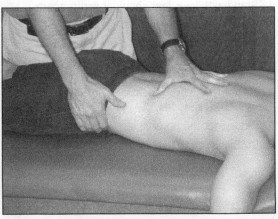

Muscle energy for restricted inhalation right rib 11

QUADRATUS LUMBORUM MUSCLE

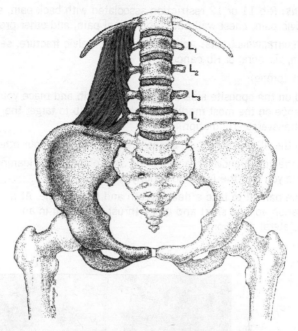

Attachments to rib 12, lumbar transverse processes, iliac crest

RIB 11–12 THRUST

INDICATIONS: Rib 11 or 12 restriction associated with back pain, sacral pain, pelvic pain, chest wall pain, abdominal pain, and other problems.

RELATIVE CONTRAINDICATIONS: Acute rib fracture, pelvic fracture, severe low back pain, vertebral or rib cancer.

TECHNIQUE (prone):

1. Stand on the opposite side of the restricted rib and place your thenar eminence on the most medial aspect of that rib to target the costotransverse articulation;

2. Grasp the ASIS on the side of the restricted rib with your other hand;

3. Push the costotransverse articulation anterolaterally by leaning onto it while you pull the ASIS posteriorly;

4. Ask the patient to take a deep breath and then exhale. At maximum exhalation apply a short and quick thrust on the rib in an anterolateral direction;

5. Retest rib motion.

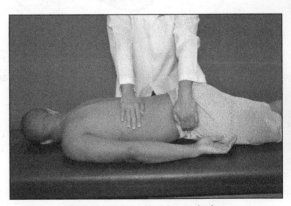

Thrust for left rib 11 restriction

9 Cervical Diagnosis and Treatment

Diagnosis of Cervical Somatic Dysfunction:
1. Screening
   Cervical range of motion *p. 196*
   Posterior cervical palpation *p. 197*
   Anterior cervical palpation *p. 198*
   Key lesion screening using compression *p. 198*
2. Motion testing
   Sidebending testing *p. 199*
   Translation testing *p. 200*
3. Cervical somatic dysfunction (Table 9-1) *p. 201*
4. Neurological exam
   Cervical compression test *p. 202*
   Vertebral artery challenge test *p. 202*

Treatment of Cervical Somatic Dysfunction:
1. OMT
   Suboccipital inhibition *p. 203*
   Cervical kneading *p. 203*
   Cervical stretching *p. 204*
   Scalene ligamentous articular strain *p. 205*
   Posterior C1 counterstrain *p. 206*
   Posterior C2–C7 counterstrain *p. 207*
   Anterior C1 counterstrain *p. 208*
   Anterior C2–C7 counterstrain *p. 209*
   Cervical myofascial release *p. 210*
   Cervical ligamentous articular strain *p. 211*
   Occipitoatlantal myofascial release *p. 212*
   Cervical soft tissue-facilitated positional release *p. 213*
   Suboccipital-facilitated oscillatory release *p. 214*
   Cervical-seated facet release *p. 215*
   Cervical long restrictor muscle energy *p. 216*
   Cervical sidebending muscle energy/thrust *p. 218*
   Cervical rotation muscle energy/thrust *p. 219*
   Cervical sidebending articulatory—supine *p. 220*
   Cervical rotation articulatory—supine *p. 221*
   Atlantoaxial muscle energy *p. 222*
   Atlantoaxial thrust *p. 223*
   Occipitoatlantal muscle energy *p. 224*
   Occipitoatlantal thrust *p. 225*
2. Exercises
   Cervical extensor stretch *p. 204*
   Scalene stretch *p. 206*
   Posterior cervical position of ease *p. 207*
   Cervical joint position of ease *p. 208*
   Sternocleidomastoid position of ease *p. 209*
   Scalene position of ease *p. 210*
   Trapezius stretch *p. 217*
   Levator stretch *p. 217*

Cervical sidebending self-mobilization *p. 220*
Sternocleidomastoid stretch *p. 223*

Diagnosis

SCREENING

Cervical Range of Motion

1. With the patient seated, observe for the following normal rays of active (patient induced) motion[1]:

   a) Flexion $\geq 50°$
   b) Extension $\geq 60°$
   c) Rotation $\geq 80°$
   d) Sidebending $\geq 45°$

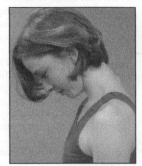

Active flexion

2. With the patient seated or supine, test the following ranges of passive (physician induced) motion, which are normally equal to or greater than active motion:

   a) Flexion
   b) Extension
   c) Rotation
   d) Sidebending

3. Restricted active and passive motion = somatic dysfunction or anatomical restriction;

4. Restricted active and normal passive motion = possible muscle weakness, fatigue, inhibition, or guarding;

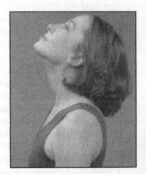

Active extension

5. Restricted passive and normal active motion = muscle guarding.

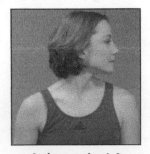

Active rotation left

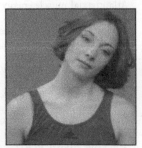

Active sidebending left

Posterior Cervical Palpation

1. Palpate for tension and tenderness in the paraspinal musculature;

2. Tender point locations:

Posterior C2–C7 midline—spinous processes;
Posterior C2–C7 lateral–posterior aspect of articular pillar at facet joint.

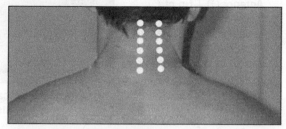

Tender point locations (left lateral points not shown)

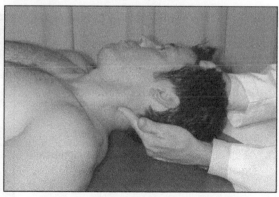

Palpation of left PC3 lateral tender point

Anterior Cervical Palpation

1. Palpate for tension and tenderness in the scalene and sternocleidomastoid muscles;

2. Palpate for the following tender points:

   Anterior C1—tip of C1 transverse process or posterior mandible angle; Anterior C2–C6—anterior aspect of articular pillar at facet joints; Anterior C7 (not shown)—lateral sternocleidomastoid muscle just superior to clavicle; Anterior C8—just superior to medial clavicle.

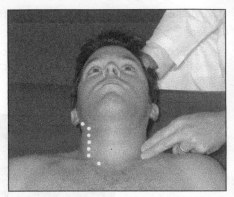

**Palpation of scalene muscles
(tender points indicated)**

Key Lesion Screening Using Compression

1. Hold the head of the seated patient with one hand and place the other hand on the lumbosacral junction;

2. Gently compress the head toward the inferior hand, assessing for ease of sidebending, rotation, and flexion-extension;

3. Vector of ease is toward the most significant somatic dysfunction.

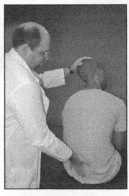

Compression using head

TYPICAL CERVICAL MOTION TESTING

Sidebending Testing

1. With the patient supine, gently hold the occiput in your palms and place your fingertips on the lateral aspects of the articular pillars of the segment with facet joint fullness;

2. Induce segmental sidebending by simultaneously bending the head to one side and pushing medially into the articular pillar on that side, comparing to the other side to identify laxity and restriction;

3. Induce segmental rotation by pushing anteriorly into the articular pillar on one side, comparing to the other side to identify laxity and restriction;

4. If restricted, retest sidebending or rotation in cervical flexion (head lifted) and extension (articular pillars lifted);

5. Restricted sidebending or rotation left = sidebending and rotation right somatic dysfunction;

   Restricted sidebending or rotation right = sidebending and rotation left somatic dysfunction;

6. Restriction worse in flexion = extension somatic dysfunction;

   Restriction worse in extension = flexion somatic dysfunction.

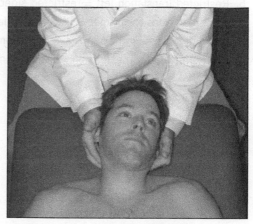

Testing C3 sidebending left

Translation Testing

1. With the patient supine, gently hold the head in your palms and place your fingertips on the lateral aspects of the articular pillars of the segment being tested (occiput for occipitoatlantal joints);

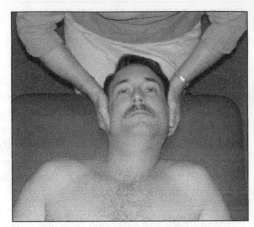

Testing occipitoatlantal translation left/sidebending right

2. Move the head and segment being tested laterally to one side to induce sidebending to the other side (e.g., translation left = sidebending right);

3. Compare to translation toward the other side to identify sidebending restriction;

4. If restricted, retest translation in cervical flexion (head lifted) and extension (articular pillars lifted);

5. Restricted translation left = restricted sidebending right;

   Restricted translation right = restricted sidebending left;

6. Restriction worse in flexion = extension somatic dysfunction;

   Restriction worse in extension = flexion somatic dysfunction.

Table 9-1 | CERVICAL SOMATIC DYSFUNCTION

Somatic Dysfunction	Diagnostic Finding
Posterior tender point	Tenderness at posterior articular pillar
Anterior tender point	Tenderness at anterior articular pillar
C2–C7 F Sx Rx	Restricted C2–C7 sidebending y and rotation y, worse in extension
C2–C7 E Sx Rx	Restricted C2–C7 sidebending y and rotation y, worse in flexion
AA Rx	Restricted C1 rotation y
OA F Sx Ry	Restricted occiput sidebending y and rotation x, worse in extension
OA E Sx Ry	Restricted occiput sidebending y and rotation x, worse in flexion

Abbreviations: F, flexion; E, extension; S, sidebending; R, rotation; x, right or left; y, left or right (opposite x); AA, atlantoaxial; OA, occipitoatlantal.

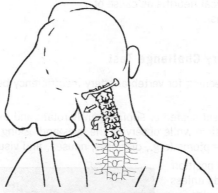

**C2–C7 sidebending and rotation left
(Drawing by William A. Kuchera, DO, FAAO)**

NEUROLOGICAL EXAM BEFORE TREATMENT

Cervical Compression Test

INDICATIONS: Neck pain radiating to the arm or associated with arm numbness, tingling, or weakness.

1. With the patient seated or supine, place your hands on top of the head and push firmly in an inferior direction without flexing or extending the neck. Variation: Add sidebending to compression;

2. Reproduction or exacerbation of arm pain, numbness, or tingling indicates possible cervical neuritis as cause of arm symptoms.

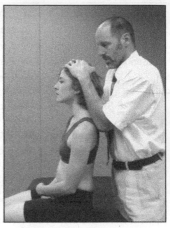
Cervical compression test

Vertebral Artery Challenge Test

INDICATIONS: Screening for vertebral artery insufficiency before cervical manipulation.

1. With the patient seated or supine, gently rotate and extend the head as far as possible while observing the eyes and asking the patient to report any symptoms (e.g., dizziness, nausea, and visual changes);

2. Maintain this position for 20 seconds unless symptoms develop;

3. Dizziness, nausea, sweating, or nystagmus in this position indicates possible vertebral artery insufficiency—avoid direct techniques;

4. If no symptoms develop, repeat with rotation to the other side.

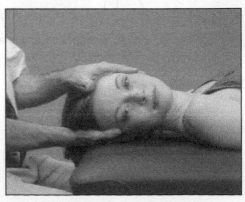
Vertebral artery challenge test

Treatment

SUBOCCIPITAL INHIBITION

INDICATIONS: Suboccipital muscle tension association with neck pain, headache, respiratory congestion, visceral dysfunction, and other problems.

RELATIVE CONTRAINDICATIONS: Atlantoaxial instability, meningismus.

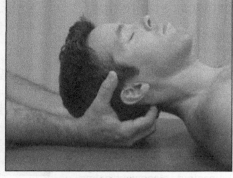

Suboccipital inhibition

TECHNIQUE (supine):

1. Hold the occiput in your palms and align your fingertips inferior to the inion;
2. Straighten your fingers to press the fingertips into the suboccipital muscles;
3. Hold this position until the muscles relax and the head drops into your palms;
4. Retest for suboccipital muscle tension.

CERVICAL KNEADING

INDICATIONS: Cervical paraspinal muscle tension associated with neck pain, headache, and other problems.

RELATIVE CONTRAINDICATIONS: Meningismus.

TECHNIQUE (supine):

1. Standing on the opposite side of muscle tension, place your cephalad hand on the forehead and use your other hand to grasp the paraspinal musculature lateral to the spinous processes;

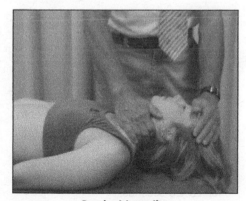

Cervical kneading

2. Slowly pull the tense muscles anteriorly without sliding over the skin, resisting head rotation with your cephalad hand;
3. Repeat kneading until tension is reduced;
4. Repeat for the other side if needed.

CERVICAL STRETCHING

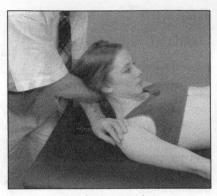

Cervical stretching

INDICATIONS: Posterior cervical muscle tension associated with neck pain, headache, upper back pain, and other problems.

RELATIVE CONTRAINDICATIONS: Acute strain and sprain, acute fracture, and meningismus.

TECHNIQUE (supine):

1. Cross your wrists under the occiput, place your palms downward on top of the shoulders, and slowly stand up to flex the neck as far as it will comfortably go. Alternative technique: hold the occiput in your palms and slowly flex the neck as far as it will comfortably go;

2. Maintain gentle force at the flexion barrier until tissue give is completed;

3. Slowly lower the head to the table and retest for muscle tension. If improved, consider prescribing CERVICAL EXTENSOR STRETCH.

CERVICAL EXTENSOR STRETCH

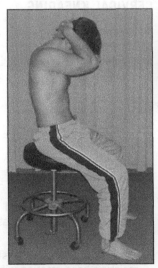

Cervical extensor stretch

1. Sit with your feet flat on the floor;

2. Place your hands on the back of the head;

3. Keeping the back straight, let the chin drop down toward the chest and allow the weight of your arms to pull the head down;

4. Take a few deep breaths and stretch for 10–20 seconds;

5. Do this stretch 1–4 times a day.

SCALENE LIGAMENTOUS ARTICULAR STRAIN

INDICATIONS: Scalene tension associated with neck pain, headache, facial pain, thoracic outlet syndrome, and other problems.

RELATIVE CONTRAINDICATIONS: Supraclavicular mass.

TECHNIQUE (supine):

1. Sit at the head of the table and place your thumb pads in the supraclavicular fossa just lateral to the sternocleidomastoid muscles;

2. Gently push your thumbs inferiorly into the anterior scalene muscles;

3. Maintain inferior pressure until tissue give is completed;

4. Gently pull your thumbs laterally, maintaining inferior and lateral pressure until tissue give is completed;

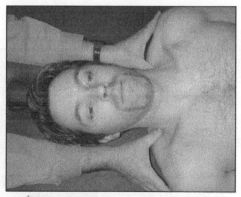

Anterior scalene ligamentous articular strain

Middle and posterior scalene ligamentous articular strain

5. Place your thumb pads just posterior to the anterior scalene position and gently push inferiorly and medially into the middle and posterior scalene muscles;

6. Maintain inferior and medial pressure until tissue give is completed;

7. Retest for scalene tension, if improved consider prescribing SCALENE STRETCH.

SCALENE STRETCH

1. While seated, hold onto the chair with one hand;
2. Hold the top of the head with your other hand;
3. Allow the head to slowly fall to the side away from the tight scalene muscles as far as it will comfortably go, letting the weight of arm move the head;
4. Take a few deep breaths and stretch for 10–20 seconds;
5. Repeat steps 3 and 4 with the head bent slightly backward;
6. Repeat these stretches for the other side;
7. Do this stretch 1–4 times a day.

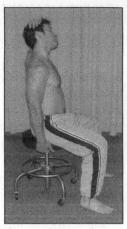

Scalene stretch

POSTERIOR C1 COUNTERSTRAIN

INDICATIONS: Posterior C1 tender point associated with neck pain, headache, and other problems.

RELATIVE CONTRAINDICATIONS: Acute cervical fracture or dislocation, vertebrobasilar insufficiency.

TECHNIQUE (supine):

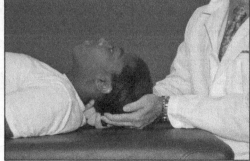

Counterstrain for right posterior C1

1. Locate the tender point just inferior to the lateral nuchal line or on the posterior arch of the atlas, labeling it 10/10;
2. Gently push the back of the head inferiorly to extend the occiput;
3. Retest for tenderness and fine-tune with slight extension, sidebending, or rotation until tenderness is minimized to 0/10 if possible but at most to 3/10;
4. Hold this position of maximum relief for 90 seconds, maintaining finger contact to monitor for tissue texture changes while reducing pressure;
5. Slowly and passively return the neck to neutral and retest for tenderness with the same pressure as initial labeling.

POSTERIOR C2–C7 COUNTERSTRAIN

INDICATIONS: Posterior C2–C7 tender point associated with neck pain, headache, and other problems.

RELATIVE CONTRAINDICATIONS: Acute fracture or dislocation, vertebrobasilar insufficiency.

TECHNIQUE (supine):

1. Locate the tender point on the spinous process or articular pillar, labeling it 10/10;

2. Extend the head and retest for tenderness;

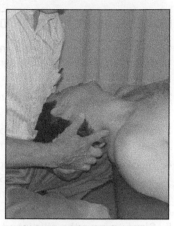

Counterstrain for right PC4 tender point

3. Fine-tune this position with slight head sidebending and rotation away from the tender point until tenderness is minimized to 0/10 if possible but at most to 3/10;

4. Hold this position of maximum relief for 90 seconds, maintaining finger contact to monitor for tissue texture changes while reducing pressure;

5. Slowly and passively return the neck to neutral and retest for tenderness with the same pressure as initial labeling. If improved, consider prescribing POSTERIOR CERVICAL POSITION OF EASE or CERVICAL JOINT POSITION OF EASE.

POSTERIOR CERVICAL POSITION OF EASE

1. Lying on your back, insert a small pillow or rolled up towel behind your neck;

2. Allow your head to drop back over the pillow and rest on the floor;

3. If comfortable, take a few deep breaths and rest in this position for 2–5 minutes if no dizziness, blurred vision, or nausea occurs;

4. Remove the pillow and roll to one side before getting up slowly;

5. Use this position 2–4 times a day or as needed for pain relief.

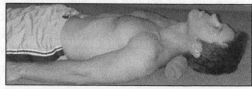

Posterior cervical position of ease

CERVICAL JOINT POSITION OF EASE

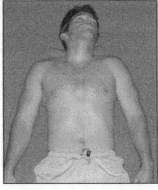

1. Lying on your back, insert a small pillow or rolled up towel under the neck;
2. Allow the head to fall back around the pillow;
3. Slowly turn the head away from the side of neck pain until it decreases;
4. If comfortable, take a few deep breaths and rest in this position for 2–5 minutes unless dizziness, blurred vision, or nausea develop;

Cervical joint position of ease

5. Slowly remove the pillow and roll to one side before getting up;
6. Use this position 2–4 times a day or as needed for pain relief.

ANTERIOR C1 COUNTERSTRAIN

INDICATIONS: Tender point at C1 transverse process associated with neck pain, headache, and other problems.

RELATIVE CONTRAINDICATIONS: Acute fracture or dislocation, atlantoaxial instability, vertebrobasilar insufficiency.

TECHNIQUE (supine):

Right anterior C1 tender point and treatment position

1. Locate the tender point at the C1 transverse process located between the angle of the mandible and the mastoid process, labeling it 10/10;
2. Rotate the head away from the tender point and retest for tenderness;
3. Fine-tune this position with more rotation and slight flexion until tenderness is minimized to 0/10 if possible but at most to 3/10;
4. Hold this position of maximum relief for 90 seconds, maintaining finger contact to monitor for tissue texture changes while reducing pressure;
5. Slowly and passively return the neck to neutral and retest for tenderness with the same pressure as initial labeling. If improved, consider prescribing STERNOCLEIDOMASTOID POSITION OF EASE.

STERNOCLEIDOMASTOID POSITION OF EASE

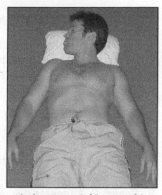
Left sternocleidomastoid position of ease

1. Lie on your back with the head resting on one or two pillows;

2. With the head bent slightly toward the side of neck pain, allow the head to rotate away from the side of pain;

3. If comfortable, take a few deep breaths and rest in this position for 2–5 minutes;

4. Slowly roll to one side before getting up;

5. Repeat 2–4 times a day or as needed for pain relief.

ANTERIOR C2–C7 COUNTERSTRAIN

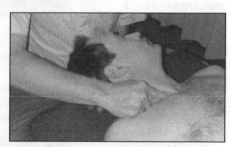
Right anterior C7 tender point and treatment position

INDICATIONS: Anterior C2–C7 tender point associated with neck pain, headache, and other problems.

RELATIVE CONTRAINDICATIONS: Acute cervical fracture or dislocation.

TECHNIQUE (supine):

1. Locate the tender point on the anterior aspect of the articular pillar, labeling it 10/10;

2. Flex the head and retest for tenderness;

3. Fine-tune this position with slight flexion, sidebending, and rotation until tenderness is minimized to 0/10 if possible but at most to 3/10:

    AC2–C6—usually sidebending and rotation away from tender point;
    AC7—usually sidebending toward and rotation away from tender point;

4. Hold this position of maximum relief for 90 seconds, maintaining finger contact to monitor for tissue texture changes while reducing pressure;

5. Slowly and passively return the neck to neutral and retest for tenderness with the same pressure as initial labeling. If improved, consider prescribing SCALENE POSITION OF EASE or STERNOCLEIDOMASTOID POSITION OF EASE.

SCALENE POSITION OF EASE

1. Lie on your back with the head resting on one or two pillows;
2. Bend the head to the side of neck pain;
3. If comfortable, take a few deep breaths and rest in this position for 2–5 minutes;
4. Slowly roll to one side before getting up;
5. Repeat 2–4 times a day or as needed for pain relief.

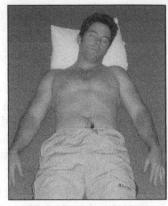

Scalene position of ease

CERVICAL MYOFASCIAL RELEASE

INDICATIONS: C2–C7 restriction related to neck pain, headache, and other problems.

RELATIVE CONTRAINDICATIONS: Acute cervical fracture, vertebral cancer.

TECHNIQUE (supine):

1. Sitting at the head of the table, hold the occiput in your palms and place your fingertips at the lateral articular pillar on both sides of the restricted segment;

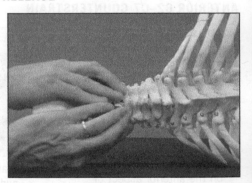

Hand position

2. Indirect: Gently move the head and restricted segment to the position of sidebending, rotation, and flexion–extension laxity and follow any tissue release until completed;
3. Direct: Slowly move the head and restricted segment into the sidebending, rotation, and flexion–extension restrictions and apply steady force until tissue give is completed;
4. Retest sidebending.

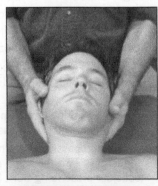

C3 myofascial release

CERVICAL LIGAMENTOUS ARTICULAR STRAIN

INDICATIONS: Cervical joint tension, tenderness, or restriction related to neck pain, headache, and other problems.

RELATIVE CONTRAINDICATIONS: Acute cervical fracture, vertebral cancer.

TECHNIQUE (supine):

1. Place your thenar eminences on the superior nuchal ridge medial to occipitomastoid sutures;
2. Place your fingertips on the articular pillars one segment below the somatic dysfunction;
3. Compress the somatic dysfunction by pushing your fingertips anteriorly and superiorly while pushing the occiput inferiorly;
4. Maintain compression until tissue give is completed;
5. Retest for joint somatic dysfunction.

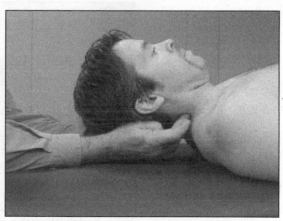

Cervical ligamentous articular strain

OCCIPITOATLANTAL MYOFASCIAL RELEASE

INDICATIONS: Restricted suboccipital fascia rotation related to neck pain, headache, upper respiratory congestion, and other problems.

RELATIVE CONTRAINDICATIONS: Acute cervical fracture.

TECHNIQUE (supine):

1. Place your fingertips on the skin in the suboccipital area and test fascial rotation right and left to identify restriction and laxity;

2. Indirect: Rotate the suboccipital fascia to its position of laxity and follow any tissue release until completed;

3. Direct: Rotate the suboccipital fascia into its restriction and apply steady force until tissue give is completed;

4. Retest suboccipital fascial rotation.

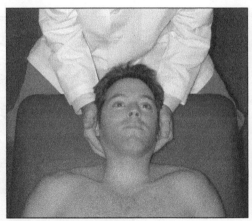

Occipitoatlantal myofascial release

CERVICAL SOFT TISSUE-FACILITATED POSITIONAL RELEASE

INDICATIONS: Cervical paraspinal tension associated with neck pain, headache, and other problems.

RELATIVE CONTRAINDICATIONS: Acute cervical fracture, vertebral cancer.

TECHNIQUE (supine):

1. Sit at the head of the table and palpate the paraspinal tension with one hand;

2. Holding the top of the head with your other hand, slowly flex the neck to reduce the cervical lordosis;

3. Slowly sidebend and rotate the head toward the paraspinal tension until it decreases;

4. Slightly extend the head until paraspinal tension is further reduced;

5. Hold this position for 3–5 seconds until tension release is completed and slowly return the head to neutral;

6. Retest for paraspinal tension.

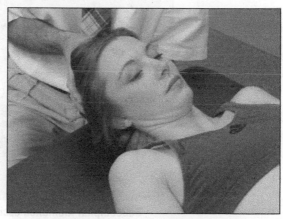

Cervical soft tissue facilitated positional release for right tension

SUBOCCIPITAL-FACILITATED OSCILLATORY RELEASE

INDICATIONS: Suboccipital tension associated with neck pain, headache, and other problems.

RELATIVE CONTRAINDICATIONS: Acute fracture, significant patient guarding.

TECHNIQUE (supine):

1. Sit at the head of the table and gently hold the occiput in your palms;

2. Use one or two fingertips to apply focal pressure to tense tissues;

3. Move the head into flexion, rotation, or sidebending to apply positional stretch to the tense tissues;

4. While stabilizing the head, add gentle oscillatory motion through your finger contact by movement of the wrist in alternately opposite directions;

5. Continue oscillation until tension is reduced.

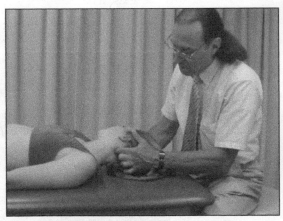

Suboccipital facilitated oscillatory release

CERVICAL SEATED FACET RELEASE

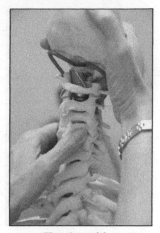

INDICATIONS: Restricted cervical motion associated with neck pain, headache, and other problems.

RELATIVE CONTRAINDICATIONS: Acute cervical sprain or fracture.

TECHNIQUE:

1. Stand behind the patient and increase upper thoracic kyphosis by flexing the head and having the patient lean back into your abdomen;

2. Place your thumb on the inferior facet of the locked open or closed facet group;

Thumb position

3. Place your other hand on the head and gently compress inferiorly while flexing the cervical spine, keeping the patient leaning against your abdomen. Repeat for the other side to determine the side of facet restriction;

4. Test the side of facet restriction for the position of greatest restriction by gentle compression and recoil on the head to close and open the locked facet;

5. Hold the patient in the position of greatest restriction and gently induce a small amount of additional compression or traction through the head to induce glide of the facet, thereby releasing the restriction;

6. Retest cervical motion.

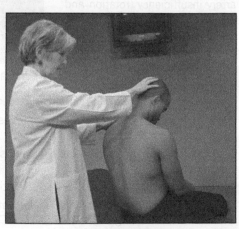

Initial positioning

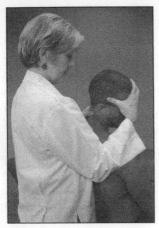

Compression for right C3

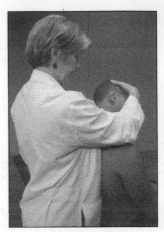

Traction for right C3

CERVICAL LONG RESTRICTOR MUSCLE ENERGY

INDICATIONS: Restricted cervical range of motion associated with neck pain, headache, upper back pain, and other problems.

RELATIVE CONTRAINDICATIONS: Acute strain and sprain, acute fracture, meningismus, cervical neuritis (sidebending only), and vertebral artery insufficiency (rotation and extension only).

TECHNIQUE (supine): See also CERVICAL STRETCHING.

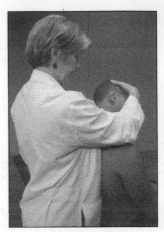

Cervical sidebending muscle energy

1. Hold the occiput in one or both hands and slowly move the cervical region to its restrictive barrier;

2. Ask the patient to push away from the restriction against your equal resistance for 3–5 seconds;

3. Allow the patient to fully relax and then slowly move head to a new restrictive barrier;

4. Repeat this contraction and stretch 3–5 times or until motion returns;

5. Slowly lower the head to the table and retest motion. If improved, consider prescribing CERVICAL EXTENSOR STRETCH, TRAPEZIUS STRETCH, or LEVATOR STRETCH.

TRAPEZIUS STRETCH

1. While sitting, hold on to the chair with one hand;

2. Hold the top of your head with the other hand;

3. Allow the head to slowly fall to the side away from the tight trapezius muscle as far as it will comfortably go, letting the weight of the arm move the head;

4. Take a few deep breaths and stretch for 10–20 seconds;

5. Repeat to the other side;

6. Do this stretch 1–4 times a day.

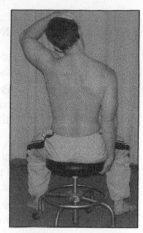

Trapezius stretch

LEVATOR STRETCH

1. While seated, hold onto the chair with one hand;

2. Hold the top of your head with the other hand with fingertips just above the opposite ear;

3. Allow the head to slowly fall first forward and then to the side away from the tight levator scapula muscle as far as it will comfortably go;

4. Take a few deep breaths and stretch for 10–20 seconds;

5. Repeat for the other side;

6. Do this stretch 1–4 times a day.

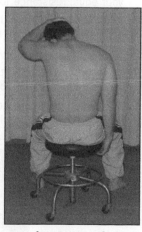

Levator stretch

CERVICAL SIDEBENDING MUSCLE ENERGY/THRUST

INDICATIONS: Restricted sidebending C2–C7 related to neck pain, headache, and other problems.

RELATIVE CONTRAINDICATIONS: Joint inflammation, acute sprain, acute fracture, undiagnosed cervical radiculopathy, vertebral artery insufficiency, and joint hypermobility (thrust only).

TECHNIQUE (supine):

1. Hold the occiput in your palms and place your index finger at the superior aspect of the restricted segment with that arm pointing toward the opposite axilla;

2. Move the head into its flexion–extension and sidebending restrictive barriers around your metacarpophalangeal joint;

3. Rotate the head away from the sidebending restriction to better localize the barrier;

4. Ask the patient to sidebend the head away from the restriction into your equal resistance for 3–5 seconds;

5. Allow the patient to fully relax and slowly move the head to a new sidebending restrictive barrier;

6. Repeat this contraction and stretch 3–5 times or until motion returns;

7. For thrust, exert a short quick sidebending movement with your metacarpophalangeal joint toward the opposite axilla;

8. Retest cervical sidebending, if improved consider prescribing CERVICAL SIDEBENDING SELF-MOBILIZATION.

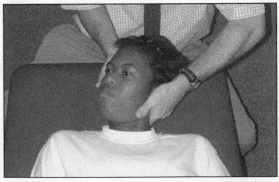

Sidebending muscle energy for C3 extended, rotated and sidebent right

CERVICAL ROTATION MUSCLE ENERGY/THRUST

INDICATIONS: Restricted rotation C2–C7 related to neck pain, headache, and other problems.

RELATIVE CONTRAINDICATIONS: Joint inflammation, acute sprain, acute fracture, undiagnosed cervical radiculopathy, vertebral artery insufficiency, and cervical joint hypermobility (thrust only).

TECHNIQUE (supine):

1. Hold the occiput in your palms and place your index finger at the superior aspect of the restricted segment with that arm pointing toward the jaw;
2. Move the head into its flexion–extension and rotation restrictive barriers around your metacarpophalangeal joint;
3. Sidebend the head away from the rotation restriction to better localize the barrier;
4. Ask the patient to rotate the head away from the restriction into your equal resistance for 3–5 seconds;
5. Allow the patient to fully relax and slowly move the head to a new rotation restrictive barrier;
6. Repeat this contraction and stretch 3–5 times or until motion returns;
7. For thrust, exert a short quick rotational movement with your metacarpophalangeal joint toward the jaw;
8. Retest cervical rotation.

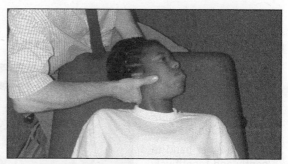

Rotational muscle energy for C3 extended, rotated and sidebent right

CERVICAL SIDEBENDING ARTICULATORY—SUPINE

INDICATIONS: Restricted sidebending C2–C7 related to neck pain, headache, and other problems.

RELATIVE CONTRAINDICATIONS: Joint inflammation, acute sprain, acute fracture, cervical joint hypermobility, undiagnosed cervical radiculopathy, vertebral cancer, and vertebral artery insufficiency.

TECHNIQUE:

1. Hold the patient's occiput in your palms;

2. Place your index finger at the superior aspect of the restricted segment and gently push toward the patient's opposite axilla;

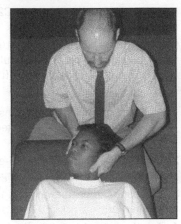

Sidebending articulatory for C3 rotated and sidebent right

3. In one smooth motion, slowly flex the head, sidebend it toward the restriction, rotate away from the restriction, and extend the head around your metacarpophalangeal joint;

4. Repeat 3–5 times or until joint mobility returns;

5. Retest cervical sidebending, if improved consider prescribing CERVICAL SIDEBENDING SELF-MOBILIZATION.

CERVICAL SIDEBENDING SELF-MOBILIZATION

1. Lie on your back and use one hand to grip both sides of the back of the neck just below the restricted area;

2. Use the other hand to gently and repetitively move the head into sidebending around the hand at the back of the neck;

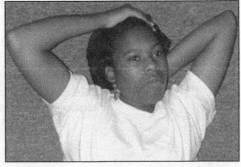

Cervical sidebending self-mobilization

3. Repeat for the other side if needed;

4. Do up to twice a day if helpful.

CERVICAL ROTATION ARTICULATORY—SUPINE

INDICATIONS: Restricted rotation C2–C7 related to neck pain, headache, and other problems.

RELATIVE CONTRAINDICATIONS: Joint inflammation, acute sprain, acute fracture, cervical joint hypermobility, undiagnosed cervical radiculopathy, vertebral cancer, and vertebral artery insufficiency.

TECHNIQUE:

1. Hold the patient's occiput in your palms;
2. Place your index finger at the superior aspect of the restricted segment and gently push toward the patient's jaw;
3. In one smooth motion, slowly flex the head, rotate it toward the restriction, sidebend away from the restriction, and extend the head around your metacarpophalangeal joint;
4. Repeat 3–5 times or until joint mobility occurs;
5. Retest cervical rotation.

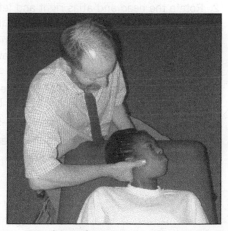

Rotation articulatory for C3 rotated and sidebent right

ATLANTOAXIAL MUSCLE ENERGY

INDICATIONS: Restricted atlantoaxial (AA) rotation related to neck pain, headache, and other problems.

RELATIVE CONTRAINDICATIONS: Acute fracture or dislocation, acute sprain, atlantoaxial instability, and verte-brobasilar insufficiency.

TECHNIQUE (supine):

AA muscle energy for restricted left rotation

1. Place your fingertips on the atlas in the suboc-cipital area and use your palms to gently lift the head to a flexion restrictive barrier;

2. Rotate the head and atlas right and left to identify a restriction, discontinuing if dizziness, nausea, diaphoresis, or nystagmus occurs;

3. Rotate the head and atlas to the rotation restrictive barrier and ask the patient to gently rotate the head away from the restriction against your equal resistance for 3–5 seconds;

4. Allow the patient to fully relax and then slowly move the head and atlas to a new rotation restrictive barrier;

5. Repeat this contraction and stretch 3–5 times or until motion returns;

6. Retest atlantoaxial rotation, if improved consider prescribing STERNOCLEIDOMASTOID STRETCH.

ATLANTOAXIAL THRUST

INDICATIONS: Restricted atlantoaxial (AA) rotation related to neck pain, headache, and other problems.

RELATIVE CONTRAINDICATIONS: Acute fracture or dislocation, acute sprain, atlantoaxial instability, and vertebrobasilar insufficiency.

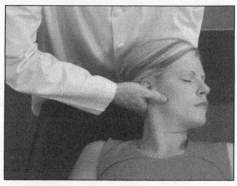
Thrust for restricted C1 rotation left

TECHNIQUE (supine):

1. Hold the occiput and gently lift the head to a flexion restrictive barrier to localize rotation to the atlas;
2. Place your first metacarpophalangeal joint on the posterior arch of the atlas and rotate the head and atlas to the rotation restrictive barrier;
3. Have the patient take a deep breath and at the end of exhalation apply a short quick movement of the atlas into the rotation restrictive barrier, avoiding rotation of the entire head;
4. Retest atlantoaxial rotation, if improved consider prescribing STERNOCLEIDOMASTOID STRETCH.

STERNOCLEIDOMASTOID STRETCH

1. Lie on your back with the head resting on a pillow;
2. Allow the head to turn to one side as far as is comfortable;
3. With one hand on the cheek, allow the weight of the arm to turn the head farther;
4. Take a few deep breaths and stretch for 10–20 seconds, stopping sooner if there is dizziness, blurred vision, or nausea;
5. Repeat to the other side;
6. Do this stretch 1–4 times a day.

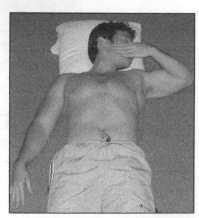
Left sternocleidomastoid stretch

OCCIPITOATLANTAL MUSCLE ENERGY

INDICATIONS: Restricted occipitoatlantal (OA) motion related to neck pain, headache, and other problems.

RELATIVE CONTRAINDICATIONS: Acute fracture or dislocation, acute sprain, atlantoaxial instability, and vertebrobasilar insufficiency.

TECHNIQUE (supine):

1. Gently sidebend or translate the occiput in neutral, flexion, and extension to identify an occipitoatlantal restriction;
2. Discontinue if dizziness, nausea, diaphoresis, or nystagmus occurs;
3. Move the occiput into its flexion–extension and sidebending restrictive barriers and ask the patient to gently sidebend the head away from the restriction against your equal resistance for 3–5 seconds;
4. Allow the patient to fully relax and then slowly move the head to a new sidebending restrictive barrier;
5. Repeat this contraction and stretch 3–5 times or until motion returns;
6. Retest occipitoatlantal motion.

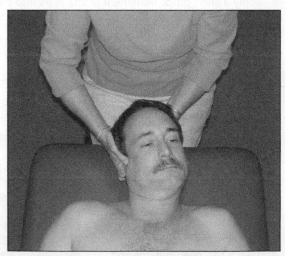

Muscle energy for OA extended, sidebent left rotated right

OCCIPITOATLANTAL THRUST

INDICATIONS: Restricted occipitoatlantal (OA) motion related to neck pain, headache, and other problems.

RELATIVE CONTRAINDICATIONS: Acute cervical fracture or sprain, atlantoaxial instability, vertebrobasilar insufficiency.

TECHNIQUE (supine):

1. Hold the occiput and gently nod the head into its flexion or extension restrictive barrier;

2. Place your first metacarpophalangeal joint on the occiput inferior to the nuchal ridge, sidebend the head to its restrictive barrier, and rotate the head away from the sidebending restriction;

3. Have the patient take a deep breath and at the end of exhalation apply a short quick movement of the occiput into the sidebending restriction;

4. Release immediately and retest occipitoatlantal motion. If still restricted apply a rotation thrust:

   a) Hold the occiput and gently nod the head into its flexion or extension restrictive barrier;

   b) Place your first metacarpophalangeal joint on the occiput inferior to the nuchal ridge, rotate the head to its restrictive barrier, and sidebend the head away from the rotation restriction;

   c) Have the patient take a deep breath and at the end of exhalation apply a short quick movement of the occiput into the rotation restriction;

   d) Release immediately and retest occipitoatlantal motion.

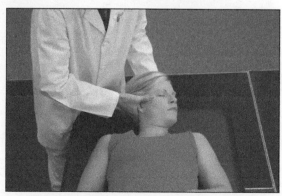

Sidebending thrust for OA extended, sidebent left rotated right

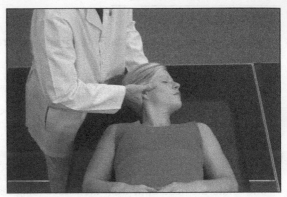

Rotation thrust for OA extended, sidebent left extended, sidebent right

REFERENCE

1. AMA. *Guides to the Evaluation of Permanent Impairment*. 4th ed. Chicago, MA: American Medical Association; 1994.

10 Head Diagnosis and Treatment

Diagnosis of Head Somatic Dysfunction:
1. Screening
   Cranial palpation *p. 228*
   Cranial motion testing *p. 230*
   Vault hold *p. 230*
   Frontooccipital hold *p. 231*
   Posterior temporal hold *p. 231*
2. Temporomandibular joint (TMJ) palpation/motion testing *p. 232*
3. Head somatic dysfunction (Table 10-1) *p. 233*
4. Sphenobasilar Synchondrosis Somatic Dysfunction (Table 10-2) *p. 234*

Treatment of Head Somatic Dysfunction:
1. OMT
   Facial efflcurage *p. 235*
   Venous sinus drainage *p. 237*
   Compression of the 4th ventricle *p 239*
   Frontal lift *p. 240*
   Parietal lift *p. 211*
   SBS compression–decompression *p. 242*
   Trigeminal stimulation *p. 243*
   Sphenopalatine ganglion stimulation *p. 245*
   Temporal decompression *p. 246*
   TMJ compression/decompression *p. 247*
   V-spread (suture disengagement) *p. 248*
   Mandibular drainage *p. 249*
   Occipital decompression *p. 250*
   Balanced membranous tension *p. 251*
2. Exercises
   Trigeminal self-stimulation *p. 244*
   TMJ self-mobilization *p. 248*
   Cervical extensor stretch see *p. 204*

Diagnosis

SCREENING

Cranial Palpation

1. Palpate the following cranial sutures for tenderness:

   Sagittal suture—midline between parietal bones;
   Coronal suture—between parietal and frontal bones;
   Bregma—juncture of sagittal and coronal sutures;
   Lambdoidal suture—between parietal bones and occiput;
   Lambda—juncture of sagittal and lambdoidal sutures;

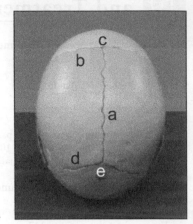

Superior cranial landmarks

   Occipitomastoid suture—between occiput and mastoid processes;
   Asterion—juncture of occiput, parietal, and temporal bones;
   Squamosal suture—between parietal and temporal bones;
   Pterion—juncture of frontal, parietal, sphenoid, and temporal bones;
   Metopic suture—midline between two halves of frontal bone in children and some adults (not shown).

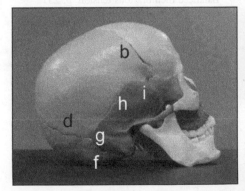

Lateral cranial landmarks

Dural Venous Sinuses

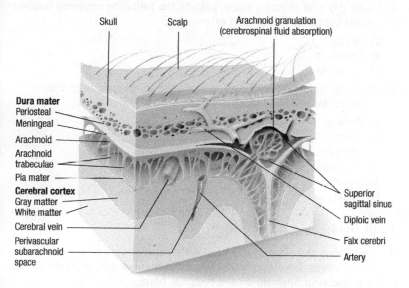

Skull   Scalp   Arachnoid granulation (cerebrospinal fluid absorption)

Dura mater
Periosteal
Meningeal
Arachnoid
Arachnoid trabeculae
Pia mater
Cerebral cortex
Gray matter
White matter
Cerebral vein
Perivascular subarachnoid space

Superior sagittal sinus
Diploic vein
Falx cerebri
Artery

Superior sagittal sinus is interior to metopic suture, sagittal suture, mid-sagittal occiput

Cranial Motion Testing

1. Using the hold of your choice, palpate the following unpaired midline cranial bones for flexion and extension:
   a) Occiput
   b) Sphenoid
   c) Mandible

2. Using the hold of your choice, palpate the following paired cranial bones for external and internal rotation:
   a) Parietal
   b) Frontal
   c) Temporal
   d) Zygoma
   e) Maxilla
   f) Nasal

Vault Hold

1. Gently hold the sides of the head with index fingers on sphenoid greater wings, third and fourth fingertips anterior and posterior to the ears, and fifth fingertip on the occipital bone;

2. Your thumbs are resting lightly on the vertex of the head;

3. Follow the cranial rhythmic impulse and evaluate for rate, amplitude, and symmetry.

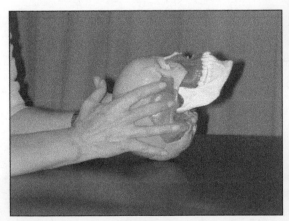

Vault hold

Frontooccipital Hold

1. Let the occiput rest in one hand, avoiding pressure on the occipitomastoid sutures;
2. Let your other hand rest on the frontal bone just above the eyebrows with the thumb on one greater wing of sphenoid and middle fingertip on the other greater wing;
3. Follow the cranial rhythmic impulse and evaluate for rate, amplitude, and symmetry.

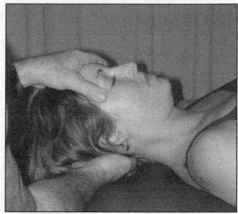

Frontooccipital hold

Posterior Temporal Hold

1. Gently hold the temporal bones with your thumbs on the sphenoid greater wings, index fingers posterior to the ears, and fifth fingertip on the squamous portion of the occipital bone;
2. Follow the cranial rhythmic impulse and evaluate for rate, amplitude, and symmetry.

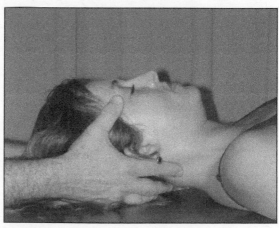

Posterior temporal hold

TEMPOROMANDIBULAR PALPATION/MOTION TESTING

1. Place your first and second fingertips at the temporomandibular (TMJ) joints located just anterior to the lower earlobes;
2. Palpate for tenderness and asymmetry;
3. Ask the patient to slowly open the mouth as far as possible;
4. The mandible normally opens symmetrically without crepitus in the joints;
5. Deviation of the mandible to one side during opening indicates TMJ restriction on that side.

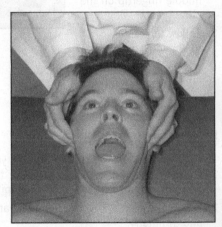

TMJ palpation and motion testing

Table 10-1 | HEAD SOMATIC DYSFUNCTION

Somatic Dysfunction	Exam Findings	Etiology
Slow rate	CRI^a rate < 10 cycles/minute	Slow metabolism Chronic infection Chronic fatigue
Fast rate	CRI rate > 14 cycles/minute	Fast metabolism Acute infection
Low amplitude	CRI amplitude < 3/5	Dural tension SBS^b compression
SBS^b torsion	Sphenoid and occiput rotate in opposite direction around an A-P axis	Postural strain Cervical dysfunction Head trauma May be normal
SBS^b sidebending rotation	Sphenoid and occiput rotate in same direction around an A-P axis and in opposite direction around parallel vertical axes	Postural strain Cervical somatic dysfunction Head trauma May be normal
SBS^b vertical strain	Sphenoid and occiput rotate in same direction around parallel transverse axes	Head trauma
SBS^b lateral strain	Sphenoid and occiput rotate in same direction around parallel vertical axes	Head trauma
SBS^b compression	Sphenoid and occiput have little or to no mobility	Head trauma Depression Severe emotional trauma
Internal rotation	Paired bone restricted in external rotation	Head trauma Dural tension
External rotation	Paired bone restricted in internal rotation	Head trauma Dural tension
TMJ dysfunction	TMJ tenderness, crepitus, and restricted opening	Myofascial strain Dental malocclusion Cranial dysfunction Joint degeneration

[a]Cranial rhythmic impulse normals: Rate = 10–14 cycles/minute; Amplitude = 3–5/5; Rhythm = symmetrical.
[b]Sphenobasilar synchondrosis at juncture of sphenoid and occiput.

Table 10-2 | SPHENOBASILAR SYNCHONDROSIS SOMATIC DYSFUNCTION

Somatic Dysfunction	Right Sphenoid Greater Wing	Left Sphenoid Greater Wing	Right Occiput	Left Occiput
Right torsion^a	Superior	Inferior	Inferior	Superior
Left torsion^a	Inferior	Superior	Superior	Inferior
Right sidebending rotation^b	Inferior and anterior	Superior and posterior	Inferior and posterior	Superior and anterior
Left sidebending rotation^b	Superior and posterior	Inferior and anterior	Superior and anterior	Inferior and posterior
Right lateral strain^c	Medial and anterior	Lateral and posterior	Lateral and anterior	Medial and posterior
Left lateral strain^c	Lateral and posterior	Medial and anterior	Medial and posterior	Lateral and anterior
Inferior vertical strain^c	Superior	Superior	Inferior	Inferior
Superior vertical strain^c	Inferior	Inferior	Superior	Superior
Compression	No motion	No motion	No motion	No motion

^{a}Torsions are named for the superior greater wing of the sphenoid.
^{b}Sidebending rotations are named for the side of head convexity.
^{c}Sphenobasilar strains are named for the direction of basisphenoid movement which is opposite to greater wing movement.

Treatment

FACIAL EFFLEURAGE

INDICATIONS: Tension headache, upper respiratory congestion, and other problems.

RELATIVE CONTRAINDICATIONS: Intracranial bleed, craniofacial fracture, central nervous system (CNS) malignancy, CNS infection, cystic acne.

TECHNIQUE (seated or supine):

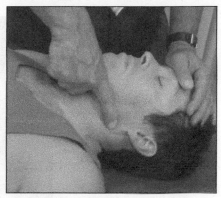

Step 1: Lateral neck effleurage

1. Place your fingertips inferior to the ears and firmly slide them inferiorly over the skin toward the medial clavicles, avoiding pressure on the carotid arteries and repeating as often as needed to facilitate lymphatic drainage;

2. Perform one or more of the following techniques, repeating as often as needed to facilitate lymphatic drainage:

   a) Place your thumbs or fingertips at the midline of the forehead and firmly slide them laterally over the skin toward the ears;

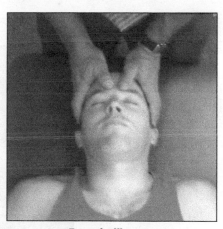

Frontal effleurage

   b) Place your thumbs or fingertips at the bridge of the nose and firmly slide them laterally over the skin toward the angles of the mandible;

   c) Place your thumbs or fingertips at the midline of the mandible and firmly slide them laterally over the skin toward the angles of the mandible.

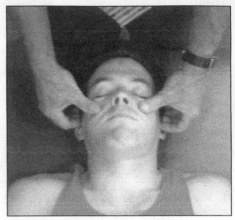

Maxilla effleurage

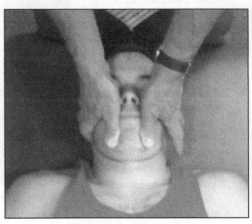

Mandible effleurage

VENOUS SINUS DRAINAGE

INDICATIONS: Headache, upper respiratory congestion, and other problems.

RELATIVE CONTRAINDICATIONS: Intracranial bleed, craniofacial fracture, central nervous system (CNS) malignancy, CNS infection.

TECHNIQUE (supine):

1. Seated at the head of the table, align your fingertips along the superior nuchal ridge with fifth fingers on the inion and exert slight superior and lateral pressure until tissue give is completed;

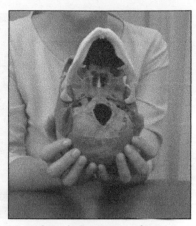

Step 1: Transverse sinus

2. Align your fingertips on both sides of the midline of the occipital bone with fifth fingers on the inion and exert slight anterior and lateral pressure until tissue give is completed;

3. Cross your thumbs and contact the opposite parietal bone on both sides of the sagittal suture at lambda, exerting slight inferior and lateral pressure until tissue give is completed and repeating anteriorly along the sagittal suture until reaching bregma;

4. Align your fingertips on both sides of the metopic suture or along the midline of the frontal bone and exert slight posterior and lateral pressure until tissue give is completed.

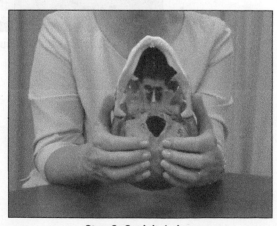

Step 2: Occipital sinus

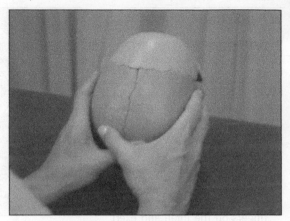

Step 3: Superior sagittal sinus

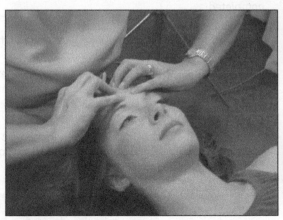

Step 4: Superior sagittal sinus at metopic suture

COMPRESSION OF THE 4TH VENTRICLE (CV4)

INDICATIONS: Diminished cranial rhythmic impulse (CRI) amplitude related to headache, upper respiratory congestion, and other problems.

RELATIVE CONTRAINDICATIONS: Intracranial bleed, craniofacial fracture, central nervous system (CNS) malignancy, CNS infection.

TECHNIQUE (supine):

1. Sit at the head of the table and place one hand on top of the other with the thenar eminences aligned;

2. Place the thenar eminences on the occipital bone inferior to the superior nuchal ridge and medial to the occipitomastoid sutures;

3. Palpate cranial flexion and extension and use your hands and intention to gently encourage extension and resist flexion until the CRI stops at a still point;

4. Maintain this extension still point until CRI flexion returns, and then gently release pressure to allow full flexion. If unable to feel the CRI, allow the occiput to rest on your hands for 1–2 minutes without exerting pressure;

5. Re-examine CRI amplitude.

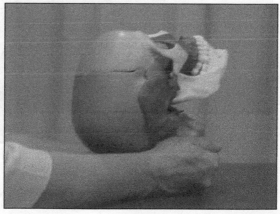

CV4

FRONTAL LIFT

INDICATIONS: Restricted frontal mobility associated with headache, depression, sinus congestion, pediatric development abnormalities, and other problems.

RELATIVE CONTRAINDICATIONS: Intracranial bleed, craniofacial fracture, central nervous system (CNS) malignancy, CNS infection.

TECHNIQUE (supine):

1. Sit at the head of the table and use your fingertips to gently contact the frontal bone posterior to the orbital ridge on both sides;
2. Palpate the cranial rhythmic impulse or gently apply anterior traction to identify restricted frontal mobility;
3. Gently lift the frontal bone anteriorly until slight give is equal on both sides;
4. Re-examine frontal mobility.

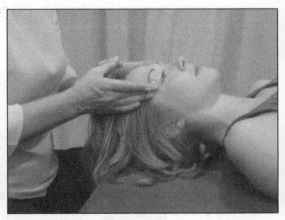

Frontal lift

PARIETAL LIFT

INDICATIONS: Restricted parietal mobility associated with headache, upper respiratory congestion, pediatric development abnormalities, and other problems.

RELATIVE CONTRAINDICATIONS: Intracranial bleed, craniofacial fracture, central nervous system (CNS) malignancy, CNS infection.

TECHNIQUE (supine):

1. Sit at the head of the table and use your fingertips to gently contact the lateral aspect of the parietal bones superior to the squamous sutures, with your thumbs crossed but off the top of the head;
2. Palpate the cranial rhythmic impulse to identify restricted parietal mobility;
3. Gently press medially into the parietal bones until slight give is equal on both sides;
4. Gently lift the parietal bones superiorly until slight give is equal on both sides;
5. Re-examine parietal mobility.

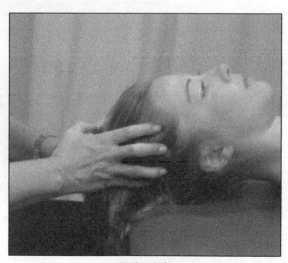

Parietal lift

SBS COMPRESSION–DECOMPRESSION

INDICATIONS: Diminished CRI amplitude related to headache, mood disorders, cranial nerve entrapment, upper respiratory congestion, pediatric development abnormalities, and other problems.

RELATIVE CONTRAINDICATIONS: Intracranial bleed, craniofacial fracture, central nervous system (CNS) malignancy, CNS infection.

TECHNIQUE (supine):

1. Using the posterior temporal or frontooccipital hold, gently compress the sphenobasilar synchondrosis (SBS) by moving the sphenoid greater wings posteroinferiorly and the occiput anterosuperiorly until slight give is equal on both sides;

2. Gently decompress the SBS by lifting the sphenoid greater wings anterosuperiorly and occiput posteroinferiorly until slight give is equal on both sides;

3. Slowly release decompression and re-examine the CRI for return of sphenoid and occiput mobility.

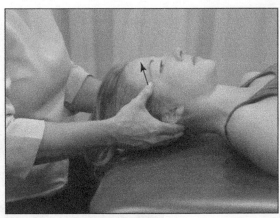

SBS decompression

TRIGEMINAL STIMULATION

INDICATIONS: Tenderness at the trigeminal foramina associated with upper respiratory congestion and other problems.

RELATIVE CONTRAINDICATIONS: Intracranial bleed, craniofacial fracture, central nervous system (CNS) malignancy, CNS infection.

TECHNIQUE (supine, seated, standing):

1. Use a finger to palpate trigeminal foramina which can be identified as a small depression at the following locations:

   Ophthalmic division (VI)—supraorbital notch on the medial supraorbital ridge;

   Maxillary division (V2)—infraorbital foramen on the medial infraorbital ridge;

   Mandibular division (V3)—mental foramen on the anterior body of the mandible;

2. Press directly into a tender trigeminal foramen with or without rotatory pressure for 10 seconds. If successful at relieving congestion, consider prescribing TRIGEMINAL SELF-STIMULATION.

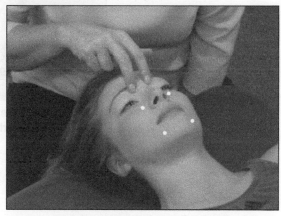

V1 stimulation (V2 and V3 marked)

TRIGEMINAL SELF-STIMULATION

1. Slide your fingertip outward along the eyebrow until you contact a tender depression in the bone;

2. Exert rotatory pressure at this depression for 10 seconds;

3. Place your fingertip at the top of the nose and slide it down along the face beside the nose until you contact a tender depression;

4. Exert rotatory pressure at this depression for 10 seconds;

5. Repeat for one or both sides as often as needed to relieve nasal congestion.

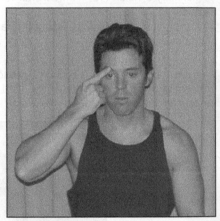

Trigeminal self-stimulation at supraorbital notch

SPHENOPALATINE GANGLION STIMULATION

INDICATIONS: Upper respiratory congestion and other problems.

RELATIVE CONTRAINDICATIONS: Intracranial bleed, craniofacial fracture, central nervous system (CNS) malignancy, CNS infection.

TECHNIQUE (supine):

1. Stand on the opposite side and insert the gloved fifth digit of your caudad hand into the mouth and along the outside of the upper molars, palpating posteriorly and then superiorly until you feel a small depression at the back roof of the mouth;

2. Exert slight pressure into this depression until tender or have the patient gently flex the head into your finger to tolerance for 3 seconds;

3. Repeat 3–5 times or until the eye starts tearing on that side;

4. Repeat on the other side if needed.

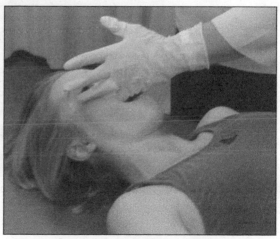

Sphenopalatine ganglion stimulation

TEMPORAL DECOMPRESSION

INDICATIONS: Restricted temporal mobility associated with headache, otitis media, vertigo, tinnitus, TMJ syndrome, and other problems.

RELATIVE CONTRAINDICATIONS: Intracranial bleed, craniofacial fracture, central nervous system (CNS) malignancy, CNS infection.

TECHNIQUE (supine):

1. Sit at the head of the table and gently grasp the posterior earlobes between your thumbs and fingertips;

2. Gently pull the ears in a posterolateral direction until slight give is equal on both sides;

3. Re-examine temporal mobility.

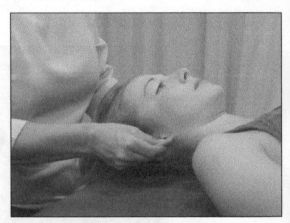

Temporal decompression

TMJ COMPRESSION/DECOMPRESSION

INDICATION: Temporomandibular joint (TMJ) restriction related to TMJ pain, mandible restriction, neck pain, and other problems.

RELATIVE CONTRAINDICATIONS: Craniofacial fracture.

TECHNIQUE (supine):

1. Sit at the head of the table and place your fingertips under the body of the mandible;

2. Gently pull the mandible superiorly toward the TMJ until slight give is equal on both sides;

3. Move your fingertips to the lateral mandible and gently push it inferiorly away from the TMJ until slight give is equal on both sides;

4. Retest TMJ mobility, if improved consider prescribing TMJ SELF-MOBILIZATION.

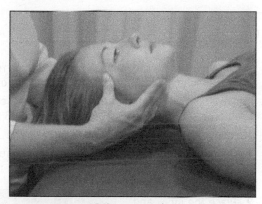

TMJ compression

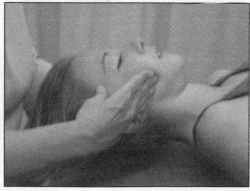

TMJ decompression

TMJ SELF-MOBILIZATION[1]

1. Place the back of the knuckles of one or two fingers inside the mouth between upper and lower teeth;

2. Gently bite down into the fingers for 5–15 seconds;

3. Repeat 2–3 times if needed;

4. Do this exercise 2–4 times a day if helpful.

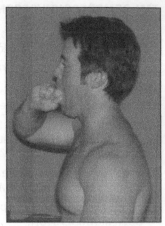

TMJ self-mobilization

V-SPREAD (suture disengagement)

INDICATIONS: Suture tenderness or cranial bone restriction associated with headache, cranial nerve entrapment, and other problems.

RELATIVE CONTRAINDICATIONS: Intracranial bleed, craniofacial fracture, central nervous system (CNS) malignancy, CNS infection.

TECHNIQUE (supine):

1. Contact the bone on either side of the suture with your index and middle finger of one hand and apply steady traction to separate the suture;

2. Place the index and middle finger of your other hand on the opposite side of the head and exert a slight repetitive impulse toward the restricted suture;

3. Continue sutural traction and contralateral impulse until sutural give is completed;

4. Retest cranial bone mobility.

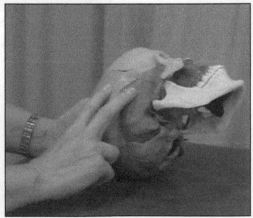

Squamous suture disengagement

MANDIBULAR DRAINAGE (Galbreath)

INDICATIONS: Otitis media, eustachian insufficiency, and other problems.

RELATIVE CONTRAINDICATIONS: Intracranial bleed, craniofacial fracture, central nervous system (CNS) malignancy, CNS infection, temporomandibular joint subluxation.

TECHNIQUE (supine):

1. Standing at one side of the head, gently hold the forehead and rotate the head toward you so the opposite eustachian tube is positioned with a downward slant toward the oropharynx;

2. Hold the angle of the opposite mandible with your fingertips;

3. Gently pull the mandible anteriorly until slight tension is encountered and then release, repeating this pull and release rhythmically for 1 minute;

4. Repeat for the other side if needed.

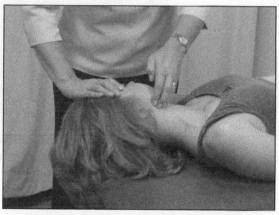

Mandibular drainage for the right eustachian tube

OCCIPITAL DECOMPRESSION

INDICATIONS: Restricted occipital mobility associated with infant feeding disorders, colic, congenital muscular torticollis, and other problems.

RELATIVE CONTRAINDICATIONS: Intracranial bleed, craniofacial fracture, central nervous system (CNS) malignancy, CNS infection.

TECHNIQUE (supine):

1. Sit at the head of the infant and gently contact the cranial base with index fingers on mastoid processes, middle fingers on occipital condyles, and ring fingers on supraocciput;

2. Gently pull the occiput in a posterior, then lateral direction while resisting mastoid process movement until slight occipital give is completed equally on both sides;

3. Re-examine occipital mobility.

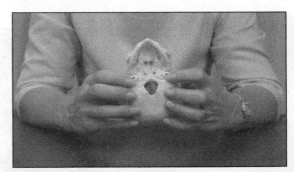

Hand placement for occipital decompression

BALANCED MEMBRANOUS TENSION

INDICATIONS: Asymmetrical or diminished cranial rhythmic impulse (CRI) related to headache, cranial nerve entrapment, and other problems.

RELATIVE CONTRAINDICATIONS: Intracranial bleed, craniofacial fracture, central nervous system (CNS) malignancy, CNS infection.

TECHNIQUE (supine):

1. Use the vault hold to palpate the CRI to identify asymmetry of motion secondary to intracranial membranous strain;

2. Indirect: Gently use your hands and intention to exaggerate membranous asymmetry;

3. Continue exaggerating membranous asymmetry and resisting return to neutral until the CRI stops at a still point;

4. Maintain this position until the CRI returns and then gently follow it back to neutral before releasing pressure;

5. Re-examine the CRI and membranes for return of symmetry.

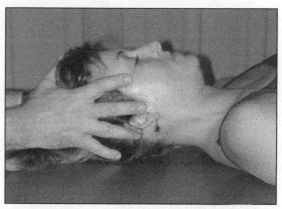

Hand position for balanced membranous tension

REFERENCE

1. Folio LR. A new osteopathic manipulative technique in homecare management of temporomandibular joint pain. *Student Doctor;* 1986:8–11.

11 Upper Extremity Diagnosis and Treatment

Diagnosis of Upper Extremity Somatic Dysfunction:

1. Screening
   Arm abduction *p. 254*
   Shoulder palpation—anterior *p. 255*
   Shoulder palpation—posterior *p. 255*
   Key lesion screening using extremities *p. 256*
2. Motion testing
   Glenohumeral abduction testing *p. 264*
   Sternoclavicular motion testing *p. 270*
   Elbow/forearm exam *p. 274*
3. Upper extremity somatic dysfunction (Table 11-1) *p. 258*
4. Neurological exam:
   Costoclavicular compression test *p. 256*
   Pectoralis minor compression test *p. 257*
   Scalene compression test *p. 257*

Treatment of Upper Extremity Somatic Dysfunction:

1. OMT
   Levator scapula counterstrain *p. 259*
   Supraspinatus counterstrain *p. 260*
   Subscapularis counterstrain *p. 261*
   Acromioclavicular counterstrain *p. 262*
   Scapula myofascial release *p. 263*
   Glenohumeral myofascial release *p. 265*
   Shoulder muscle energy *p. 266*
   Glenohumeral articulatory *p. 269*
   Clavicle muscle energy *p. 271*
   Sternoclavicular muscle energy *p. 272*
   Sternoclavicular thrust *p. 273*
   Elbow myofascial release *p. 275*
   Elbow percussion vibrator *p. 276*
   Ulna articulatory *p. 277*
   Radial head counterstrain *p. 278*
   Radial head thrust *p. 279*
   Interosseous membrane soft tissue release *p. 281*
   Forearm muscle energy *p. 282*
   Wrist counterstrain *p. 283*
   Wrist myofascial release *p. 284*
   Carpal tunnel myofascial release *p. 285*
   Wrist muscle energy *p. 286*
   Wrist articulatory *p. 287*
   First carpal–metacarpal counterstrain *p. 288*
   Carpal articulatory *p. 289*
   Upper extremity-facilitated oscillatory release *p. 290*
   Thumb metacarpal thrust *p. 290*
   Interphalangeal articulatory *p. 291*

252

2. Exercises
   Shoulder abductor position of ease *p. 261*
   Shoulder abductor stretch *p. 268*
   Shoulder self-mobilization *p. 270*
   Radial head self-mobilization *p. 280*
   Wrist extensor position of ease *p. 284*
   Carpal tunnel stretch *p. 285*
   Wrist extensor stretch *p. 287*
   Scalene position of ease *p. 210*
   Scalene stretch *p. 206*
   Rib 1 self-mobilization *p. 179*
   Pectoralis stretch *p. 191*

Diagnosis

SCREENING

Arm Abduction

1. Have the standing patient slowly abduct both arms as far as possible, keeping the palms turned outward as the hands reach above the head;

2. Observe symmetry and amount of abduction (normal = 180°). Common causes of restricted abduction: shoulder problems, elbow problems, and forearm problems;

3. Observe inferior angle of scapula rotation relative to shoulder abduction (normal scapulohumeral rhythm = 1° scapula rotation for every 2° humeral abduction). Decreased scapula rotation = shoulder girdle problem. Decreased humeral abduction = shoulder joint problem.

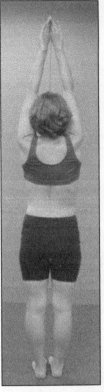

Arm abduction 180°

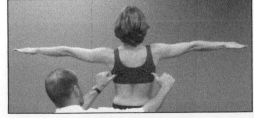

Scapulohumeral rhythm

Shoulder Palpation—Anterior

With the patient seated or supine, palpate the following structures for tenderness:

1. Sternoclavicular joint;

2. Coracoid process—inferior to lateral clavicle, pectoralis minor insertion;

3. Acromioclavicular joint;

   Subacromial bursa anterior and inferior to acromion with shoulder extension;

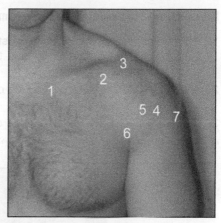

Locations of anterior shoulder tenderness

4. Greater tuberosity of humerus—inferior to acromion, supraspinatus insertion;

5. Lesser tuberosity of humerus—medial to greater tuberosity, subscapularis insertion;

   Bicipital groove between greater and lesser tuberosity;

6. Glenohumeral joint line;

7. Deltoid bursa.

Shoulder Palpation—Posterior

With the patient seated or prone, palpate the following structures for tenderness or tension:

1. Levator scapula muscle;

2. Upper trapezius muscle;

3. Supraspinatus muscle;

4. Infraspinatus muscle;

5. Posterior axillary fold—teres minor, subscapularis, and latissimus dorsi muscles;

6. Rhomboid muscle;

7. Glenohumeral joint line.

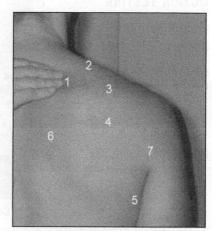

Locations of posterior shoulder tenderness

Key Lesion Screening Using Extremities

1. With the patient supine, hold the wrists or ankles and slowly move the arms or legs first to one side and then to the other side to assess ease of sidebending;
2. Hold the arms or legs in the position of sidebending ease and apply gentle traction by leaning backward;
3. Follow any tissue give to the position of maximum laxity;
4. Vector of ease is toward the most significant somatic dysfunction.

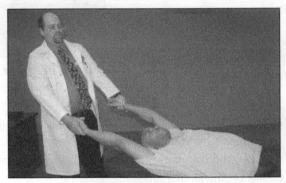

Key lesion screening using arms

MOTION TESTING

Costoclavicular Compression Test

INDICATIONS: Arm pain, numbness, or tingling.

1. Hold the wrist of the involved arm and palpate the radial pulse;
2. Ask the patient to sit up straight and use your hand and body weight to slowly push the clavicle posteroinferiorly;

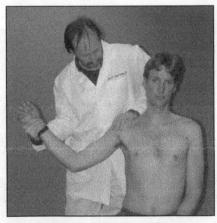

Costoclavicular compression test

3. Diminished pulse and reproduction or exacerbation of arm pain, numbness, or tingling indicate probable thoracic outlet syndrome from compression of the brachial plexus between clavicle and first rib.

Pectoralis Minor Compression Test

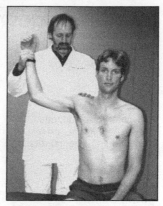

INDICATIONS: Arm pain, numbness, or tingling.

1. With the patient seated or supine, palpate the radial pulse;
2. Passively extend and abduct the shoulder to its motion barrier to stretch the pectoralis minor muscle;
3. Diminished pulse and reproduction or exacerbation of arm pain, numbness, or tingling indicate probable thoracic outlet syndrome from pectoralis minor tendon compression of the brachial plexus.

Pectoralis compression test

Scalene Compression Test (Adson maneuver)

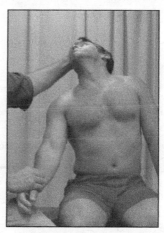

INDICATIONS: Arm pain, numbness, or tingling.

1. Palpate the radial pulse, ask the patient to take a deep breath and hold it, and bend the head backward and rotate toward the side of the radial pulse being tested;
2. Diminished pulse and reproduction or exacerbation of arm pain, numbness, or tingling indicate probable thoracic outlet syndrome from compression of the brachial plexus between anterior and middle scalene muscles.

Scalene compression test

Table 11-1 | UPPER EXTREMITY SOMATIC DYSFUNCTION

Somatic Dysfunction (position of laxity)	Diagnostic Finding
Tender points	Tender point at described location
Scapula	Restricted elevation, depression, protraction, retraction, and upward and downward rotation
Glenohumeral adduction, abduction, flexion, extension, and internal and external rotation	Restricted opposite motion
Clavicle superior	Restricted inferior glide at sternoclavicular (SC) joint with upward shoulder shrug
Clavicle inferior	Restricted superior glide at SC joint with downward shoulder shrug
Clavicle anterior	Restricted posterior glide at SC joint with forward shoulder shrug
Ulna abduction	Restricted adduction (lateral glide) at humeroulnar joint
Ulna adduction	Restricted abduction (medial glide) at humeroulnar joint
Forearm supination, pronation	Restricted opposite motion
Radial head posterior	Restricted anterior glide with supination
Radial head anterior	Restricted posterior glide with pronation
Wrist abduction, adduction, flexion, and extension	Restricted opposite motion
Metacarpal flexion, extension, abduction, and adduction	Restricted opposite motion
Interphalangeal flexion, extension, abduction, and adduction	Restricted opposite motion

Treatment

LEVATOR SCAPULA COUNTERSTRAIN

INDICATIONS: Levator scapula tender point associated with shoulder pain, arm pain, back pain, neck pain, headache, and other problems.

RELATIVE CONTRAINDICATIONS: Acute shoulder fracture or dislocation.

TECHNIQUE (lateral):

1. Locate the tender point on the superior angle of the scapula, labeling it 10/10;
2. Hook the elbow with your other arm and grasp the inferior angle of the scapula;
3. Slowly extend the shoulder and retract the scapula;
4. Retest for tenderness and fine-tune with scapula movement or compression until tenderness is minimized to 0/10 if possible but at most to 3/10;
5. Hold this position of maximum relief for 90 seconds, maintaining finger contact to monitor for tissue texture changes but reducing pressure;
6. Slowly and passively return the arm to neutral and retest for tenderness with the same pressure as initial labeling;
7. Retreat if not improved.

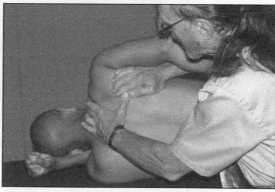

Counterstrain for right levator scapula tender point

SUPRASPINATUS COUNTERSTRAIN

INDICATIONS: Tender point in supraspinatus muscle or tendon associated with shoulder pain, arm pain, back pain, and other problems.

RELATIVE CONTRAINDICATIONS: Acute shoulder fracture or dislocation.

TECHNIQUE (supine or lateral):

1. Locate the tender point in the supraspinatus muscle or its insertion onto the greater tuberosity of the humerus, labeling it 10/10;

2. Use your other hand to slowly abduct the arm about 45° and retest for tenderness;

3. Fine-tune this position with slight arm external rotation until tenderness is minimized to 0/10 if possible but at most to 3/10;

4. Hold this position of maximum relief for 90 seconds, maintaining finger contact to monitor for tissue texture changes but reducing pressure;

5. Slowly and passively return the arm to neutral and retest for tenderness with the same pressure as initial labeling. If improved, consider prescribing SHOULDER ABDUCTOR POSITION OF EASE.

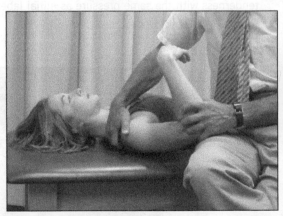

Supraspinatus counterstrain

SHOULDER ABDUCTOR POSITION OF EASE

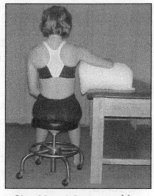

1. Sit with the involved arm resting on a table or counter;
2. Place one or two pillows under your arm;
3. If comfortable, take a few deep breaths and rest in this position for 2–5 minutes;
4. Repeat 2–4 times a day or as needed for pain relief.

Shoulder abductor position of ease

SUBSCAPULARIS COUNTERSTRAIN

INDICATIONS: Subscapularis tender point is associated with shoulder pain, arm pain, back pain, and other problems.

RELATIVE CONTRAINDICATIONS: Acute shoulder fracture or dislocation.

TECHNIQUE (supine):

1. Locate the tender point on the anterolateral scapula, labeling it 10/10;
2. Hold the distal humerus and slowly extend, internally rotate, and slightly abduct the shoulder;
3. Retest for tenderness and fine-tune with slight shoulder movements until tenderness is minimized to 0/10 if possible but at most to 3/10;
4. Hold this position of maximum relief for 90 seconds, maintaining finger contact to monitor for tissue texture changes but reducing pressure;
5. Slowly and passively return the arm to neutral and retest for tenderness with the same pressure as initial labeling.

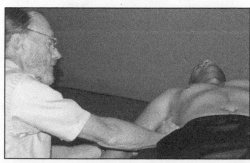

Counterstrain for right subscapularis tender point

ACROMIOCLAVICULAR COUNTERSTRAIN

INDICATIONS: Tender point at the acromioclavicular joint associated with shoulder pain, arm pain, and other problems.

RELATIVE CONTRAINDICATIONS: Acute shoulder sprain, dislocation, or fracture.

TECHNIQUE (supine):

1. Locate the tender point at the anterior acromioclavicular joint, labeling it 10/10;

2. Hold the wrist, flex and adduct the shoulder, and apply slight traction down the arm;

3. Retest for tenderness;

4. Fine-tune this position with slight changes in adduction and traction until tenderness is minimized to 0/10 if possible but at most to 3/10;

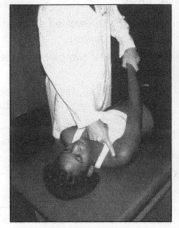

Acromioclavicular counterstrain

5. Hold this position of maximum relief for 90 seconds, maintaining finger contact to monitor for tissue texture changes but reducing pressure;

6. Slowly and passively return the arm to neutral and retest for tenderness with the same pressure as initial labeling.

SCAPULA MYOFASCIAL RELEASE

INDICATIONS: Scapula restriction or tension related to shoulder pain, arm pain, back pain, chest wall pain, and other problems.

RELATIVE CONTRAINDICATIONS: Acute scapula fracture.

TECHNIQUE (lateral):

1. Stand facing the patient and drape the involved arm over your caudad hand, which is holding the inferior angle of the scapula;

2. Hold the acromion and superior scapula with your other hand;

3. Slowly move the scapula into elevation–depression, retraction–protraction, and upward–downward rotation, determining directions of laxity and restriction;

4. Indirect: Slowly move the scapula into its positions of laxity and follow any tissue release until completed;

5. Direct: Slowly move the scapula into its restrictions and apply steady force until tissue give is completed;

6. Slowly return to neutral and retest scapula motion.

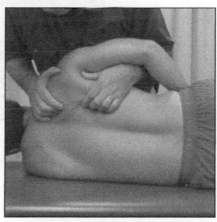

Scapula myofascial release

GLENOHUMERAL ABDUCTION TESTING

1. With the patient seated, grasp one or both arms at the elbow and induce passive abduction;

2. Restricted abduction can be due to restriction at the glenohumeral or acromioclavicular joint, tension in the scapula, latissimus dorsi or pectoralis muscles, and shoulder pain-causing muscle guarding with movement.

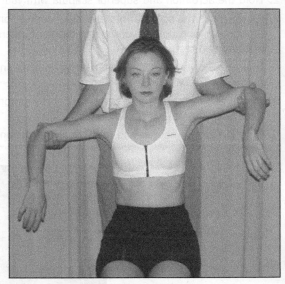

Restricted right shoulder abduction

GLENOHUMERAL MYOFASCIAL RELEASE

INDICATIONS: Glenohumeral joint restriction related to shoulder pain, arm pain, and other problems.

RELATIVE CONTRAINDICATIONS: Acute shoulder sprain or fracture, glenohumeral joint inflammation, or glenohumeral dislocation.

TECHNIQUE (supine):

1. Sit at the head of the table and firmly hold the acromioclavicular joint with one hand and the proximal forearm with your other hand;

2. Slowly abduct the arm while maintaining internal rotation, holding steady force at any restriction until tissue give is completed;

3. Slowly and externally rotate the arm and move it into additional abduction, maintaining steady force at any restriction until tissue give is completed;

4. Slowly adduct the arm while maintaining external rotation, holding steady force at any restriction until tissue give is completed;

5. Slowly return the arm to the table and retest glenohumeral motion.

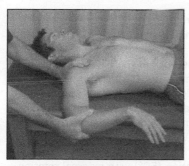
Abduction

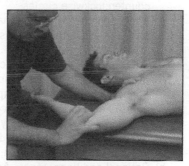
External rotation

SHOULDER MUSCLE ENERGY (Spencer Technique)

INDICATIONS: Restricted shoulder motion related to shoulder pain, adhesive capsulitis, arm pain, back pain, chest wall pain, and other problems.

RELATIVE CONTRAINDICATIONS: Acute fracture or dislocation, acute sprain, or glenohumeral joint inflammation.

TECHNIQUE (lying on opposite side):

1. Stand in front of the patient and use your cephalad hand to stabilize the acromioclavicular joint;

2. Use your other hand to test the following shoulder motions (normal range of passive motion):

   a) Extension (50°)—move the elbow posteriorly and slightly laterally;

   b) Flexion (180°)—move the elbow anteriorly and slightly medially;

   c) Circumduction with compression (smooth)—lift the elbow to about 90° abduction, compress the elbow toward the shoulder joint, and move the elbow in small clockwise and counterclockwise circles;

   d) Circumduction with traction (smooth)—lift the elbow or pull the wrist away from the shoulder joint and induce small clockwise and counterclockwise circles;

   e) Abduction (90° when internally rotated, 180° when externally rotated)—place the patient's hand on your cephalad forearm and lift the elbow laterally;

   f) Internal rotation (90°)—place the back of the patient's hand behind his or her hip and pull the elbow anteriorly;

   g) Abduction with traction (lymphatic pump)—interlock your fingertips over the deltoid muscle, place the patient's hand on your shoulder, and slowly pull the arm away from the shoulder and release, repeating 5–10 times if needed. Variation: effleurage can be applied with the same hand position;

   h) Optional additional stage: Adduction (50°) with external rotation (90°)—place the patient's hand on your cephalad forearm and move the elbow medially across the chest;

3. If a restriction is encountered, slowly move the shoulder into the barrier and ask the patient to gently push away from the restriction against your equal resistance for 3–5 seconds;

4. Allow the patient to fully relax and then slowly move the shoulder to a new restrictive barrier;

5. Repeat this contraction and stretch 3–5 times or until motion returns;

6. Retest shoulder motion, if improved consider prescribing SHOULDER ABDUCTOR STRETCH.

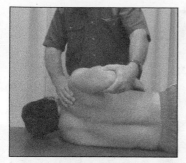

(a) Extension

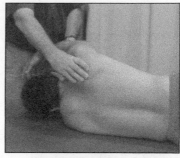

(b) Flexion

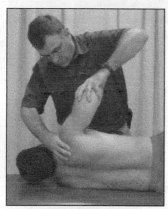

(c) Circumduction/compression

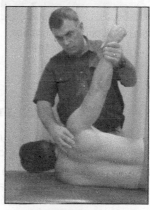

(d) Circumduction/traction

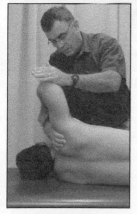

(e) Abduction

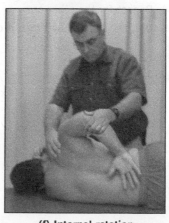

(f) Internal rotation

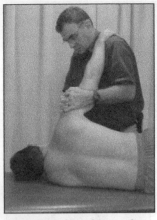
(g) Abduction with traction
(lymphatic pump)

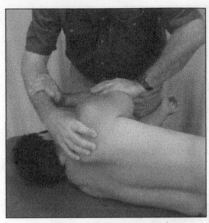
(h) Adduction/external rotation

SHOULDER ABDUCTOR STRETCH

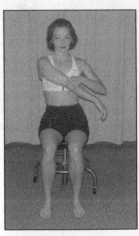

1. Grasp the involved arm just above the elbow with the other hand;
2. Allow the involved arm to relax and use the other hand to pull it across the chest as far as it will comfortably go;
3. Take a few deep breaths and stretch for 10–20 seconds;
4. Repeat for the other arm;
5. Do this stretch 2–4 times a day.

Shoulder abductor stretch

GLENOHUMERAL ARTICULATORY

INDICATIONS: Glenohumeral joint restriction related to shoulder pain and other problems.

RELATIVE CONTRAINDICATIONS: Acute shoulder sprain or fracture, glenohumeral joint hypermobility or inflammation.

TECHNIQUE (seated):

1. Stand behind the patient and firmly hold the acromioclavicular joint with one hand;

2. Grasp the wrist with your other hand and move the shoulder in an internal rotation and adduction barrier behind the patient's back;

3. Maintain the internal rotation barrier and slowly abduct the arm;

4. Maintain the abduction barrier and slowly externally rotate at the shoulder;

5. Slowly move the shoulder into flexion, adduction, and internal rotation barriers in an overhand throwing motion;

6. Repeat as one smooth motion 3–5 times or until joint mobility returns;

7. Retest glenohumeral motion, if improved consider prescribing SHOULDER SELF-MOBILIZATION.

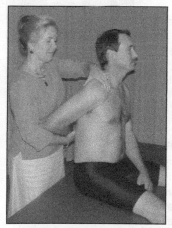

Adduction and internal rotation

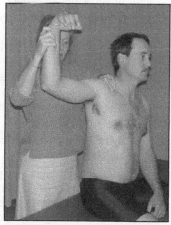

Abduction and external rotation

SHOULDER SELF-MOBILIZATION

1. Sit or stand with a 12–16 ounce can in the hand of the involved arm and the other arm leaning against a table or wall;

2. Allow the arm to hang freely and move the hand in small circles for 1–2 minutes;

3. Move the hand in small circles in the opposite direction for 1–2 minutes;

4. Do this mobilization 2–4 times a day.

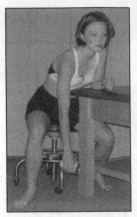

Shoulder self-mobilization

STERNOCLAVICULAR MOTION TESTING

1. With the patient seated or supine, palpate the sternoclavicular joint and ask the patient to shrug the shoulders:

   a) Superiorly to induce inferior clavicle glide;

   b) Inferiorly to induce superior clavicle glide;

   c) Anteriorly to induce posterior clavicle glide;

   d) Posteriorly to induce anterior clavicle glide;

2. Identify restrictions by comparing clavicle glide on both sides:

   Restricted inferior glide = superior clavicle;
   Restricted superior glide = inferior clavicle;
   Restricted posterior glide = anterior clavicle;
   Restricted anterior glide = posterior clavicle.

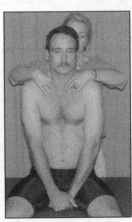

Testing inferior glide

CLAVICLE MUSCLE ENERGY

INDICATIONS: Sternoclavicular joint restriction related to shoulder pain, chest wall pain, neck pain, and other problems.

RELATIVE CONTRAINDICATIONS: Acute clavicle fracture, sternoclavicular joint inflammation, acute shoulder sprain or fracture, or glenohumeral joint hypermobility or inflammation.

TECHNIQUE (seated):

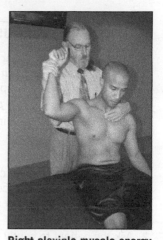
Right clavicle muscle energy

1. Stand behind the patient, hold the wrist on the side of restriction with one hand, and monitor the sternoclavicular joint with your other hand;

2. Abduct the shoulder to about 90° and externally rotate to its restrictive barrier;

3. Ask the patient to gently push the shoulder into internal rotation against your equal resistance for 3–5 seconds;

4. Allow the patient to fully relax and then slowly externally rotate the shoulder to a new restrictive barrier;

5. Repeat this contraction and stretch 3–5 times or until motion returns;

6. Retest sternoclavicular motion.

STERNOCLAVICULAR MUSCLE ENERGY

INDICATIONS: Sternoclavicular joint restriction related to shoulder pain, chest wall pain, neck pain, and other problems.

RELATIVE CONTRAINDICATIONS: Acute clavicle fracture, sternoclavicular joint inflammation.

TECHNIQUE (supine):

1. Push or pull the medial clavicle into its restrictive barrier (exception—for superior glide restriction stabilize the opposite sternoclavicular joint);

2. Ask the patient to gently contract a muscle against your equal resistance for 3–5 seconds:

   a) Anterior clavicle—patient's flexed arm pulls posteriorly into your shoulder;

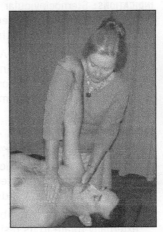

Muscle energy for right anterior clavicle

   b) Superior clavicle—patient's internally rotated arm pushes anteriorly;

   c) Inferior clavicle—patient's head rotated toward the restricted SC joint pushes into rotation away from the restricted joint;

3. Repeat 3–5 times or until motion returns;

4. Retest sternoclavicular motion.

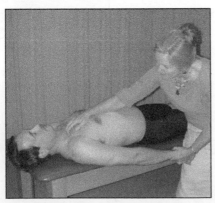

Muscle energy for right superior clavicle

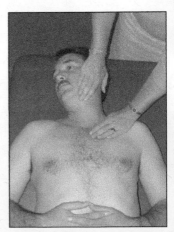

Muscle energy for right inferior clavicle

STERNOCLAVICULAR THRUST

INDICATIONS: Clavicle restricted posterior or inferior glide related to shoulder pain, chest wall pain, neck pain, and other problems.

RELATIVE CONTRAINDICATIONS: Acute clavicle fracture or dislocation, acute shoulder sprain, or sternoclavicular joint inflammation.

TECHNIQUE (supine):

1. Stand on the opposite side and place the thenar eminence of your cephalad hand on the medial clavicle, pushing it in the direction of glide restriction;

2. Gap the sternoclavicular joint by placing your caudad hand on the table between the involved arm and ribs and having the patient use the other hand to pull the wrist around your forearm toward the opposite shoulder;

3. Apply a short and quick thrust into the glide restriction with your thenar eminence;

4. Retest sternoclavicular motion.

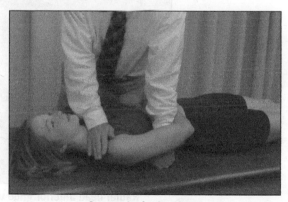

Sternoclavicular thrust

ELBOW/FOREARM EXAMINATION

1. Palpate for tenderness at the olecranon process, medial epicondyle, lateral epicondyle, and radial head. Radial head tender points are located at the anterolateral or posterolateral aspect of the radial head;

2. Palpate for tension and tenderness of the wrist flexors distal to the medial epicondyle, wrist extensors distal to the lateral epicondyle, and interosseous membrane between ulna and radius;

3. Test elbow flexion and extension to determine directions of laxity and restriction;

4. Test forearm pronation/radial head posterior glide and supination/radial head anterior glide to determine directions of laxity and restriction:

   Restricted anterior glide with supination = posterior radial head;
   Restricted posterior glide with pronation = anterior radial head.

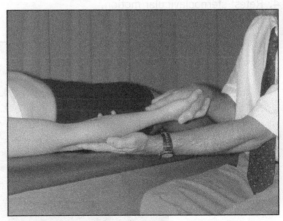

Radial head anterior glide with supination

ELBOW MYOFASCIAL RELEASE

INDICATIONS: Ulna restriction related to arm pain and other problems.

RELATIVE CONTRAINDICATIONS: Elbow joint inflammation (direct myofascial release only).

TECHNIQUE (seated or supine):

1. Hold the patient's hand with one hand and the proximal radius and ulna with your other hand;

2. Test elbow flexion–extension and forearm supination–pronation to determine directions of laxity and restriction;

3. Indirect: Gently and slowly move the elbow to its position of laxity, apply compression or traction between your hands to facilitate laxity, and follow any tissue release until it is completed;

4. Direct: Slowly move the elbow into its restriction and apply steady force until tissue give is completed;

5. Slowly return the elbow to neutral and retest motion.

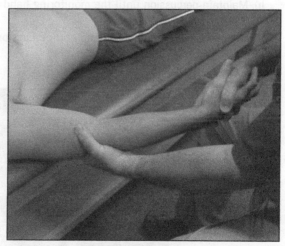

Elbow myofascial release

ELBOW PERCUSSION VIBRATOR

INDICATIONS: Ulna, radial head, or forearm somatic dysfunction associated with arm pain, elbow or forearm restriction, and other problems.

RELATIVE CONTRAINDICATIONS: Acute elbow sprain, elbow joint inflammation, upper extremity cancer, or recent elbow surgery.

TECHNIQUE (supine):

1. Place your monitoring hand over the medial epicondyle;

2. Place the vibrating percussion pad lightly on the lateral epicondyle or the radial head avoiding pad bouncing;

3. Alter pad speed, pressure, and angle until vibrations are palpated as strong by the monitoring hand;

4. Maintain contact until the force and rhythm of vibration returns to that of normal tissue;

5. Alternative technique:

   a) Allow the monitoring hand to be pulled toward the pad, resisting any other direction of hand pull;

   b) Maintain percussion until the monitoring hand is pushed away from the pad;

6. Slowly release the monitoring hand and percussion vibrator and retest motion.

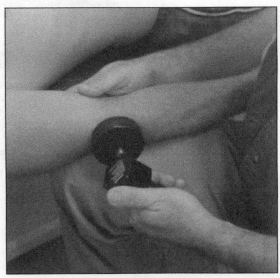

Elbow percussion vibrator

ULNA ARTICULATORY

INDICATIONS: Ulna restriction related to arm pain and other problems.

RELATIVE CONTRAINDICATIONS: Elbow inflammation, acute elbow sprain, acute fracture, or elbow joint hypermobility.

TECHNIQUE (seated or supine):

1. Hold the proximal forearm with both hands, pinning the patient's hand between your arm and ribs;

2. Flex the elbow and move the ulna to a lateral glide barrier as you slowly extend the elbow;

3. Flex the elbow again and move the ulna to a medial glide barrier as you slowly extend the elbow;

4. Repeat 3–5 times or until joint mobility returns;

5. Retest elbow extension.

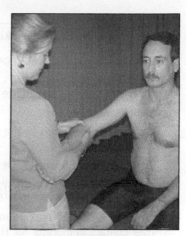

Elbow articulatory into lateral glide

RADIAL HEAD COUNTERSTRAIN

INDICATIONS: Radial head tender point associated with arm pain, forearm restriction, and other problems.

RELATIVE CONTRAINDICATIONS: Acute radius fracture.

TECHNIQUE (seated or supine):

1. Locate the tender point at the anterolateral or posterolateral head of the radius, labeling it 10/10;

2. Extend the elbow, supinate the forearm fully, and retest for tenderness;

3. Fine-tune this position with slight ulna abduction or adduction until tenderness is minimized to 0/10 if possible but at most to 3/10;

4. Hold this position of maximum relief for 90 seconds, maintaining finger contact to monitor for tissue texture changes but reducing pressure;

5. Slowly and passively return the hand to neutral and retest for tenderness with the same pressure as initial labeling;

6. Retreat if not improved.

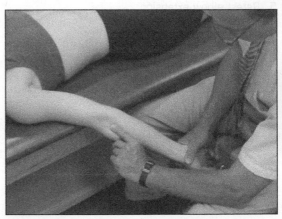

Anterior radial head tender point and treatment position

RADIAL HEAD THRUST

INDICATIONS: Restricted anterior glide of radial head associated with arm pain, forearm restriction, and other problems.

RELATIVE CONTRAINDICATIONS: Acute sprain, acute fracture, or joint inflammation.

TECHNIQUE (standing, seated, or supine):

1. Hold the patient's hand and place the thumb or thenar eminence of your other hand on the posterior aspect of the radial head;

2. Gently flex the elbow and partially pronate the hand;

3. Simultaneously extend the elbow, supinate the hand, and push the radial head anteriorly to the restrictive barriers;

4. Add a short quick anterior thrust into the radial head;

5. Retest radial head motion, if improved consider prescribing RADIAL HEAD SELF-MOBILIZATION.

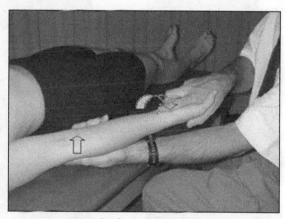

Radial head thrust

RADIAL HEAD SELF-MOBILIZATION

1. Stand with the involved elbow flexed and your fist facing the upper chest;
2. Rapidly extend the elbow as far as it will go by throwing the hand forward as you simultaneously turn the fist to face upward;
3. Repeat 2–3 times if needed;
4. Do up to twice a day.

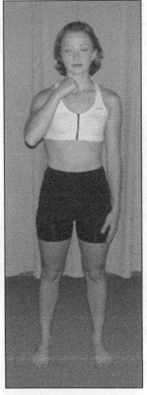

Flexion with pronation

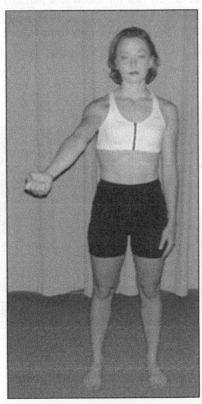

Extension with supination

INTEROSSEOUS MEMBRANE SOFT TISSUE RELEASE

INDICATIONS: Interosseous membrane tension related to arm pain, forearm restriction, and other problems. The technique can be adapted for leg interosseous membrane tension related to leg pain, ankle restriction, and other problems.

RELATIVE CONTRAINDICATIONS: Acute sprain, acute fracture, or deep venous thrombosis.

TECHNIQUE (seated or supine):

1. Palpate for tension along the ventral interosseous membrane between radius and ulna;

2. Place your thumbs over the tense area and fingers on the dorsal forearm;

3. Compress your thumbs firmly toward your fingers, adding compression or traction between your hands until tissue relaxation is completed;

4. Retest interosseous tension.

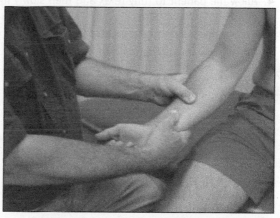

Interosseous membrane soft tissue release

FOREARM MUSCLE ENERGY

INDICATIONS: Restricted forearm supination or pronation associated with arm pain and other problems.

RELATIVE CONTRAINDICATIONS: Acute sprain, acute fracture.

TECHNIQUE (seated or supine):

1. Stabilize the affected elbow with one hand;

2. Hold the affected hand with your other hand and move the forearm to the restrictive barrier;

3. Ask the patient to gently turn the forearm away from the restriction against your equal resistance for 3–5 seconds;

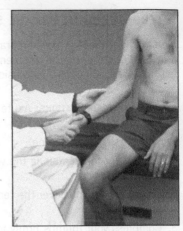

Muscle energy for restricted supination

4. Allow the patient to fully relax and then slowly move the forearm to a new restrictive barrier;

5. Repeat this contraction and stretch 3–5 times or until motion returns;

6. Retest forearm supination and pronation.

WRIST COUNTERSTRAIN

INDICATIONS: Wrist flexor or extensor tender point associated with arm pain, wrist restriction, carpal tunnel syndrome, and other problems.

RELATIVE CONTRAINDICATIONS: Acute wrist fracture.

TECHNIQUE (supine):

1. Locate the tender point at distal forearm or in the muscle belly, labeling it 10/10;

2. With the elbow on the table flex the wrist for a flexor tender point or extend the wrist for an extensor tender point;

3. Retest for tenderness and fine-tune with slight abduction or adduction until tenderness is minimized to 0/10 if possible but at most to 3/10;

4. Hold this position of maximum relief for 90 seconds, maintaining finger contact to monitor for tissue texture changes but reducing pressure;

5. Slowly and passively return the wrist to neutral and retest for tenderness with the same pressure as initial labeling. If improved, consider prescribing WRIST EXTENSOR POSITION OF EASE.

6. Retreat if not improved.

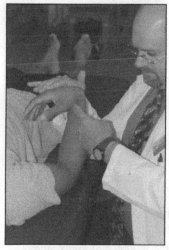

Right flexor counterstrain

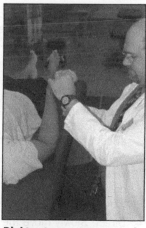

Right extensor counterstrain

WRIST EXTENSOR POSITION OF EASE

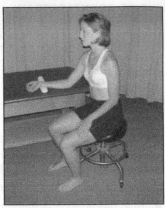

1. Sit with the involved arm resting on a table or counter and your palm facing upward;

2. Place a small pillow or rolled up towel under the wrist and allow your hand to fall back over it;

3. If comfortable, take a few deep breaths and rest in this position for 2–5 minutes;

4. Repeat 2–4 times a day or as needed for pain relief.

Wrist extensor position of ease

WRIST MYOFASCIAL RELEASE

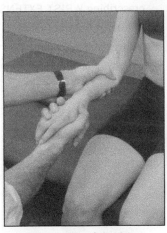

INDICATIONS: Wrist restriction related to arm pain and other problems.

RELATIVE CONTRAINDICATIONS: Acute sprain.

TECHNIQUE (seated or supine):

1. Hold the patient's forearm with one hand and his or her hand with your other hand;

2. Test wrist abduction–adduction and flexion–extension, comparing to the other hand if needed to identify directions of laxity and restriction;

Wrist myofascial release

3. Indirect: Gently and slowly move the wrist to its position of laxity, apply compression or traction between your hands to facilitate laxity, and follow any tissue release until it is completed;

4. Direct: Slowly move the wrist into its restrictions and apply steady force until tissue give is completed;

5. Slowly return the wrist to neutral and retest motion, if improved consider prescribing WRIST EXTENSOR STRETCH.

CARPAL TUNNEL MYOFASCIAL RELEASE

INDICATIONS: Carpal tunnel syndrome.

RELATIVE CONTRAINDICATIONS: Acute wrist sprain, wrist inflammation.

TECHNIQUE (seated or supine):

1. Hold the thumb with one hand and medial wrist with your other hand, placing your thumbs on the pisiform bone and hook of the hamate;

2. Slowly and externally rotate and abduct the patient's thumb, extend the wrist, and apply steady traction between your thumbs for 5 seconds;

3. Slowly release and repeat 5–15 times. If successful at reducing symptoms consider prescribing CARPAL TUNNEL STRETCH.

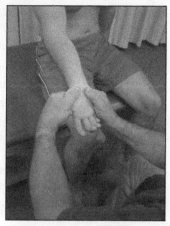

Carpal tunnel release

CARPAL TUNNEL STRETCH[1]

1. Place your palm against a wall with the fingers pointing downward;

2. With your other hand, gently pull the thumb away from the wall;

3. Gently lean into the wall to extend the wrist as far as possible;

4. If comfortable, take a few deep breaths and stretch for 10–20 seconds;

5. Repeat for the other hand;

6. Do this stretch 2–4 times a day.

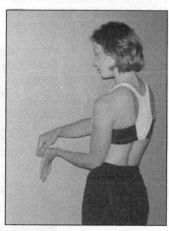

Carpal tunnel stretch

WRIST MUSCLE ENERGY

INDICATIONS: Wrist restriction related to arm pain, carpal tunnel syndrome, lateral epicondylitis, and other problems.

RELATIVE CONTRAINDICATIONS: Acute wrist fracture or sprain.

TECHNIQUE (seated or supine):

1. Hold the forearm with one hand and the hand with your other hand;
2. Test wrist flexion–extension and abduction–adduction, comparing to the other hand if needed to identify directions of restriction;
3. Slowly move the wrist to its restrictive barrier for all planes of restriction;
4. Ask the patient to gently push the hand away from the restrictive barrier against your equal resistance for 3–5 seconds;
5. Allow the patient to fully relax and then slowly move the hand to a new restrictive barrier;
6. Repeat this contraction and stretch 3–5 times or until motion returns;
7. Retest wrist motion, if improved consider prescribing WRIST EXTENSOR STRETCH.

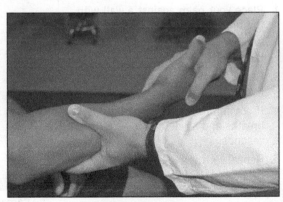

Right-wrist muscle energy

WRIST EXTENSOR STRETCH

1. Sit with the involved elbow resting on a pillow, arm straight, and hand hanging off the table with the palm facing downward;
2. Use your other hand to slowly bend the wrist downward as far as it will comfortably go;
3. Take a few deep breaths and stretch for 10–20 seconds;
4. Do this stretch 2–4 times a day.

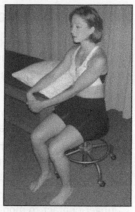

Wrist extensor stretch

WRIST ARTICULATORY

INDICATIONS: Wrist restriction related to arm pain, hand pain, and other problems.

RELATIVE CONTRAINDICATIONS: Acute sprain, wrist joint hypermobility or inflammation.

TECHNIQUE (seated or supine):

1. Grasp the sides of the patient's hand with both your hands and test flexion–extension and abduction–adduction to identify restrictions;
2. Apply traction to the wrist by leaning slowly backward until the arm is straight and the wrist joint is gapped;
3. Slowly move the wrist into its position of laxity and then into its restriction while maintaining traction;
4. Repeat 3–5 times or until joint motion returns;
5. Retest wrist motion.

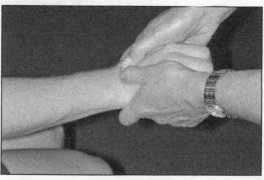

Wrist articulatory

FIRST CARPAL–METACARPAL COUNTERSTRAIN

INDICATIONS: First carpal–metacarpal tender point associated with hand pain, thumb weakness, and other problems.

RELATIVE CONTRAINDICATIONS: Acute wrist fracture.

TECHNIQUE (supine):

1. Locate the tender point on the palmar surface of the proximal first metacarpal bone, labeling it 10/10;

2. Flex and adduct the thumb and retest for tenderness, fine tuning with slightly more flexion and adduction until tenderness is minimized to 0/10 if possible but at most to 3/10;

3. Hold this position of maximum relief for 90 seconds, maintaining finger contact to monitor for tissue texture changes but reducing pressure;

4. Slowly and passively return the hand to neutral and retest for tenderness with the same pressure as initial labeling;

5. Retreat if not improved.

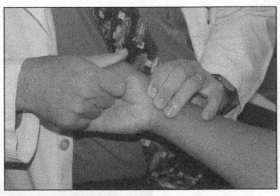

Counterstrain for right 1st carpal–metacarpal

CARPAL ARTICULATORY

INDICATIONS: Wrist restriction associated with wrist pain, hand pain, and other problems.

RELATIVE CONTRAINDICATIONS: Acute fracture or sprain, intercarpal joint inflammation.

TECHNIQUE (seated, supine, and standing):

1. Grasp the wrist with both hands with your fingers interlocked and thenar or hypothenar eminences on either side of the restricted carpal bones;

2. Ask the patient to squeeze your hand, use your thenar or hypothenar eminences to compress the carpal bones, and have the patient stop squeezing;

3. Slowly circumduct the wrist clockwise and counterclockwise 3–5 times or until motion returns;

4. Repeat for other restricted carpal bones;

5. Retest wrist motion.

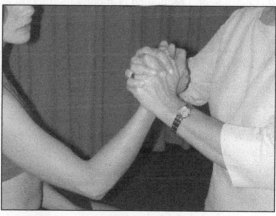

Carpal articulatory

UPPER EXTREMITY-FACILITATED OSCILLATORY RELEASE

INDICATIONS: Upper extremity somatic dysfunction associated with arm pain, restricted movement, or other problems.

RELATIVE CONTRAINDICATIONS: Acute fracture, significant patient guarding.

TECHNIQUE (supine):

1. Hold the involved arm at the hand and elbow;

2. Separate your hands to apply linear or spiral stretch to the fascia to engage a barrier;

3. Initiate horizontal or vertical oscillatory motion to the arm, feeling for restricted mobility;

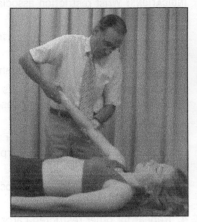

Upper extremity-facilitated oscillatory release

4. Continue arm oscillation or modify its traction and force until you feel mobility is improved.

THUMB METACARPAL THRUST

INDICATIONS: Restricted first metacarpal abduction associated with wrist pain, hand pain, and other problems.

RELATIVE CONTRAINDICATIONS: Acute sprain, carpal–metacarpal joint hypermobility or inflammation.

TECHNIQUE (seated or supine):

1. Grasp the thumb with the tip of your thumb just distal to the first carpal–metacarpal joint;

2. Use your other hand to stabilize the patient's hand;

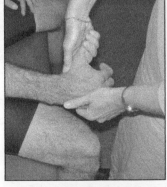

First metacarpal thrust

3. Pull the metacarpal bone distally to apply traction and abduct the thumb to its restrictive barrier;

4. Apply a short and quick abduction thrust while levering the proximal metacarpal medially with your thumb;

5. Retest first metacarpal abduction.

INTERPHALANGEAL ARTICULATORY

INDICATIONS: Interphalangeal restriction associated with hand pain and other related problems.

RELATIVE CONTRAINDICATIONS: Acute fracture or sprain, interphalangeal joint hypermobility or inflammation.

TECHNIQUE (seated or supine):

1. Stabilize the proximal bone of the joint being treated with one hand;

2. Grasp the distal bone with your other hand and gently flex and extend it to identify motion restriction;

3. Apply traction to the distal bone and slowly circumduct it in both directions 3–5 times or until motion returns;

4. Retest interphalangeal motion.

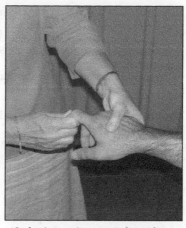

Articulatory for second proximal interphalangeal joint

REFERENCE

1. Adapted from Sucher BM. Palpatory diagnosis and manipulative management of carpal tunnel syndrome. *J Am Osteopath Assoc.* 1994;94(8):647–663.

12 Visceral Diagnosis and Treatment

Diagnosis

Table 12-1	VISCEROSOMATIC REFLEXES	
Exam	Acute Findings	Chronic Findings
Temperature	Hot	Cool
Tissue texture	Moisture, fullness, edema, tension	Thickness, dryness, ropiness, pimples
Red reflex	Increased or prolonged redness	Prolonged blanching

THORACOLUMBAR TEMPERATURE

1. With the patient seated or prone, hold your hand 1–2" posterior to the upper thoracic spine and slowly move it inferiorly along the spine to the upper lumbar area, noting variations in temperature;

2. Increased heat = possible acute somatic dysfunction;

3. Decreased heat or coolness = possible chronic somatic dysfunction.

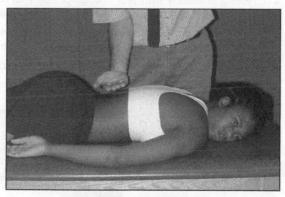

Thoracolumbar temperature

THORACOLUMBAR TISSUE TEXTURE

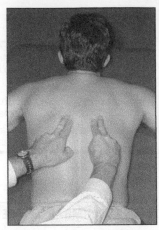

1. With the patient seated or prone, use your fingertips to palpate the thoracic and lumbar paraspinal areas from T1– L3, comparing right and left sides for skin thickness, moisture, skin drag, tension, ropiness, edema, pimples, and tenderness;

2. Moisture, fullness, edema, tension, and focal tenderness = acute somatic dysfunction;

3. Thick skin, dryness, ropiness, pimples, and ache = chronic somatic dysfunction.

Mid-thoracic tension palpation

THORACOLUMBAR RED REFLEX

1. With the patient seated or prone, place your index and middle fingers along either side of the T1 spinous process;

2. Pressing anteriorly with just enough pressure to blanch the skin, drag your fingers along the spine to the lower lumbar area;

3. Allow a few seconds for flushing to develop and note variations in the redness pattern and in the length of time different areas remain red;

4. Increased or prolonged redness = acute somatic dysfunction;

5. Prolonged blanching = chronic somatic dysfunction.

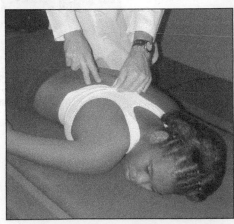

Acute upper thoracic somatic dysfunction

Table 12-2 | VISCERAL AUTONOMIC INNERVATION[a]

Organs	Sympathetic	Parasympathetic
Head and neck	T1–T4	Vagus
Cardiovascular	T1–T5	Vagus
Respiratory	T2–T7	Vagus
Stomach, liver, gall bladder	T5–T9	Vagus
Small intestines	T9–T11	Vagus
Ovaries, testicles	T9–T10	S2–S4
Kidney, ureters, bladder	T10–T11	S2–S4
Large intestines, rectum	T8–L2	Vagus—ascending colon, S2–S4—rest of colon
Uterus	T10–T11	S2–S4
Prostate	L1–L2	S2–S4

[a]From Willard FH. Autonomic nervous system. In: Ward RC, ed. *Foundations for Osteopathic Medicine*. 2nd ed. Philadelphia, PA: Lippincott Williams & Wilkins; 2003:90–119.

Vagus Nerve in Cervical Region

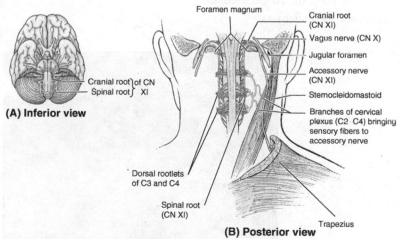

(A) Inferior view

(B) Posterior view

The vagus nerve exits jugular foramen with accessory nerve

CHAPMAN POINT PALPATION

INDICATIONS: Chest wall pain, abdominal pain, thigh pain, or visceral dysfunction.

1. Palpate for anterior Chapman points that are small tender nodules at the locations listed in the table and figures on subsequent pages;
2. Correlate the Chapman point with structural and visceral exam results;
3. If indicated, treat the associated posterior Chapman point with rotatory pressure for 1–30 seconds.

Treatment

CHAPMAN POINT STIMULATION

INDICATIONS: Chapman point tenderness related to visceral dysfunction.

RELATIVE CONTRAINDICATIONS: Bowel obstruction for intestinal points.

TECHNIQUE (seated, prone, supine, or lateral):

1. Identify a tender Chapman point by anterior or posterior palpation;
2. Use your index finger or thumb to apply rotatory pressure into the tender point for 10–30 seconds;
3. Retest for tenderness.

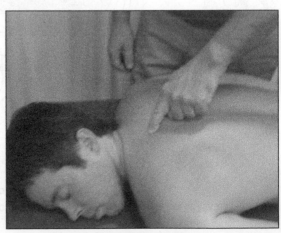

Stimulation of lower lung Chapman point

Table 12-3 | CHAPMAN POINT LOCATIONS[a]

Organ	Anterior Point	Posterior Point
Middle ear	Superior to medial clavicles	C1 posterior rami
Sinuses	Inferior to medial clavicles	C2 articular pillars
Pharynx	Inferior to sternoclavicular joints	C2 articular pillars
Tonsils	Medial 1st intercostal spaces	C2 articular pillars
Tongue	Medial 2nd ribs	C2 articular pillars
Esophagus, thyroid, heart	Medial 2nd intercostal	T2 transverse processes
Upper lung, arm	Medial 3rd intercostal	T3 transverse processes
Lower lung	Medial 4th intercostal spaces	T4 transverse processes
Liver	Right medial 5th and 6th intercostal spaces	Right T5 and T6 transverse processes
Stomach acidity	Left medial 5th intercostal space	Left T5 transverse process
Gall bladder	Right medial 6th intercostal space	Right T6 transverse process
Pancreas	Right medial 7th intercostal space	Right T7 transverse process
Spleen	Left medial 7th intercostal space	Left T7 transverse process
Small intestine	Medial 8th–10th intercostal spaces	T8–T10 transverse processes
Pyloris	Midline body of sternum	T9 transverse processes
Adrenals	1" lateral and 2" superior to umbilicus	T11 transverse processes
Kidneys	1" lateral and 1" superior to umbilicus	L1 transverse processes
Bladder	Periumbilical	L2 transverse processes
Intestine peristalsis	1–2" inferior and lateral to ASIS	Between T10 and T11 transverse processes
Appendix	Tip of rib 12	Right T11 transverse process
Ovaries	Pubic tubercles	T10 transverse processes
Urethra	Pubic tubercles	L3 transverse processes
Uterus	Inferior pubic rami	L5 transverse processes
Rectum	Lesser trochanters	Lateral aspect of middle sacrum
Colon	Anterior iliotibial bands	L2–L4 transverse processes
Prostate, broad ligament	Lateral iliotibial bands	PSIS

[a]From Patriquin DA. Chapman Reflexes. In: Ward RC, ed. *Foundations for Osteopathic Medicine*. 2nd ed. Philadelphia, PA: Lippincott Williams & Wilkins; 2003:1051–1055.

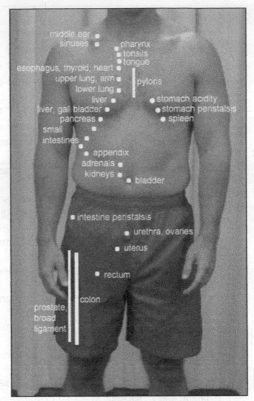

Anterior Chapman points
(points bilateral unless specified in table 12-3)

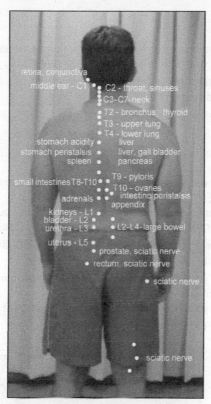

retina, conjunctiva
middle ear - C1
C2 - throat, sinuses
C3-C7-neck
T2 - bronchus, thyroid
T3 - upper lung
T4 - lower lung
liver
stomach acidity
stomach peristalsis
liver, gall bladder
spleen
pancreas
small intestines T8-T10
T9 - pyloris
T10 - ovaries
intestine peristalsis
adrenals
appendix
kidneys - L1
bladder - L2
urethra - L3
L2-L4-large bowel
uterus - L5
prostate, sciatic nerve
rectum, sciatic nerve
sciatic nerve

sciatic nerve

**Posterior Chapman points (points
bilateral unless specified in table 12-3)**

RIB RAISING

INDICATIONS: Rib restriction or organ dysfunction associated with sympathetic imbalance (see SYMPATHETIC CHAIN GANGLIA, *p. 302*).

RELATIVE CONTRAINDICATIONS: Acute rib fracture, unstable cardiac arrhythmia, or bowel obstruction.

TECHNIQUE (supine, seated):

1. Contact the rib angles with the fingertips of both hands:

   Supine from side—reach under the arm to contact rib angles on one side;
   Supine from head—reach under the shoulders to contact rib angles on both sides;
   Seated—patient's crossed arms are draped across your shoulders, reach under arms to contact rib angles on both sides;

2. Gently push or pull the rib angles anteriorly for 20–30 seconds or repetitively until rib mobility improves:

   Supine—lean your elbows into the table while keeping the wrists straight to facilitate rib lift;
   Seated—lean your body backward to facilitate rib lift;

3. Repeat for all of ribs 2–12 if needed.

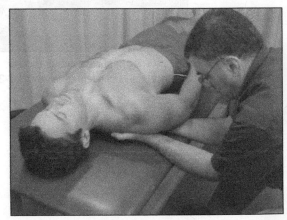

Rib raising from side

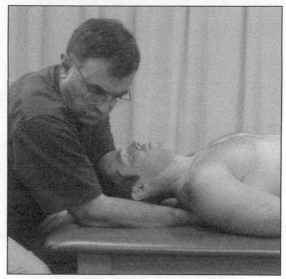

Rib raising from head (hand placement)

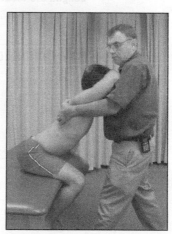

Rib raising when seated

SYMPATHETIC CHAIN GANGLIA

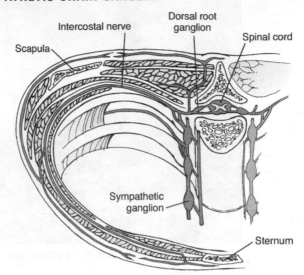

Ganglia are located anterior to rib heads

THORACOLUMBAR INHIBITION

INDICATIONS: Thoracolumbar paraspinal tension associated with abdominal or pelvic disorders.

RELATIVE CONTRAINDICATIONS: Bowel obstruction or ectopic pregnancy.

TECHNIQUE (supine):

1. Sit on the side of the tension and align your fingers under the tense paraspinal muscles with fingertips just lateral to the spinous processes;

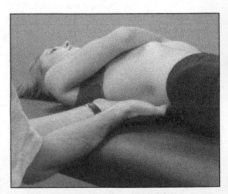

Thoracolumbar inhibition

2. Gently pull the muscles in an anterior and lateral direction by pushing your elbows downward;

3. Maintain anterior and lateral pull on the muscles until tension is reduced;

4. Repeat for the other side if needed.

SACROILIAC GAPPING

INDICATION: Sacroiliac restriction is associated with back pain, pelvic pain, hip pain, abdominal pain, constipation, diarrhea, delayed labor, and other problems.

RELATIVE CONTRAINDICATIONS: Acute pelvis fracture, sacroiliac joint inflammation, severe hip arthritis, bowel obstruction, premature labor, placenta previa, or placenta abruption.

TECHNIQUE (supine):

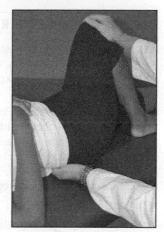

Right sacroiliac gapping

1. Stand on the side of the restriction and flex the knee and hip, placing the foot on the table close to the buttocks;
2. Pull the PSIS laterally as you gently and repetitively medially adduct the thigh to the restrictive barrier or apply lateral muscle energy isometric contraction;
3. Repeat 3–5 times or until motion returns;
4. Retest sacroiliac motion, if improved consider prescribing PELVIC TILT or SACROILIAC SELF-MOBILIZATION.

ABDOMINAL PLEXUS RELEASE

INDICATIONS: Constipation, diarrhea, gastroesophageal reflux, cholestasis, and other functional motility problems.

RELATIVE CONTRAINDICATIONS: Peritonitis, acute pancreatitis, active peptic ulcer, abdominal aortic aneurysm, bowel obstruction, recent abdominal surgery, or late pregnancy.

TECHNIQUE (supine):

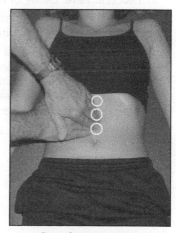

Superior mesenteric plexus release

1. Align your fingertips from just below the xiphoid process to the umbilicus;
2. Gently press into the upper (celiac plexus), middle (superior mesenteric plexus), and lower (inferior mesenteric plexus) areas to identify tension;
3. Exert steady posterior pressure into a tense area until tension releases;
4. Retest for plexus tension.

ABDOMINAL SPHINCTER RELEASE

INDICATIONS: Constipation, gastroesophageal reflux, cholestasis, and other motility problems related to sphincter tension.

RELATIVE CONTRAINDICATIONS: Peritonitis, appendicitis, acute cholecystitis, acute hepatitis, acute pancreatitis, splenomegaly, abdominal aortic aneurysm, bowel obstruction, recent abdominal surgery, or late pregnancy.

TECHNIQUE (supine):

Ileocecal valve release

1. Use your fingertips to gently push posteriorly and then clockwise and counterclockwise over the following sphincters to identify the direction of rotational ease and restriction:

   a) Pyloric sphincter: Epigastric area;
   b) Hepatopancreatic duct: Center of right upper quadrant;
   c) Duodenojejunal flexure: Center of left upper quadrant;
   d) Ileocecal valve: Center of right lower quadrant.

2. Treat the dysfunctional sphincter that has rotation opposite other sphincters with indirect or direct myofascial release;

   a) Indirect: Rotate the fascia to its position of laxity and follow any tissue release until completed;
   b) Direct: Rotate the fascia into its restriction and apply steady force until tissue give is completed;
   c) Retest fascial rotation over the dysfunctional sphincter.

LARGE INTESTINE LIFT

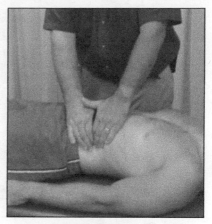

Descending colon lift

INDICATIONS: Constipation, irritable bowel syndrome, and other functional disorders.

RELATIVE CONTRAINDICATIONS: Peritonitis, colon obstruction, or recent abdominal surgery.

TECHNIQUE (supine):

1. Stand on the opposite side of the part of the colon being treated;

2. Reach across with the fingers of both hands and contact the lateral margin of the colon:

   Descending colon—left anterior axillary line;
   Transverse colon—above the umbilicus;
   Ascending colon—right anterior axillary line;

3. Gently lean backward to pull the colon toward its position of laxity:

   Descending and ascending colon—pull toward umbilicus;
   Transverse colon—pull toward epigastric area or umbilicus, whichever induces laxity;

4. Maintain the position of laxity and follow any tissue release until completed;

5. Gently return the colon to neutral.

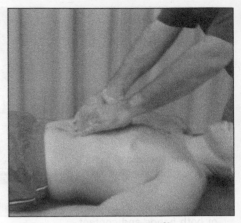

Transverse colon lift

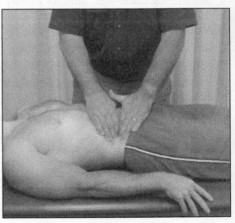

Ascending colon lift

SMALL INTESTINE LIFT

INDICATIONS: Indigestion, delayed gastric emptying, cholestasis, and other functional disorders.

RELATIVE CONTRAINDICATIONS: Peritonitis, splenomegaly, or recent abdominal surgery.

TECHNIQUE (supine):

1. Stand to the right side of the patient, reach across with the fingers of both hands, and contact the lateral margin of the small intestine near the midclavicular line in the left lower quadrant;

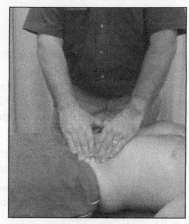

Small intestine lift

2. Gently lean backward to pull the small intestine superomedially toward the umbilicus to its position of laxity;

3. Follow any tissue release until completed;

4. Gently return the small intestine to neutral.

THORACIC PUMP

INDICATIONS: Atelectasis, bronchitis, pneumonia, peripheral edema, and other problems.

RELATIVE CONTRAINDICATIONS: Acute rib fracture, severe osteoporosis, aspiration, lung cancer, pulmonary embolism, acute congestive heart failure, peritonitis, or recent abdominal surgery.

TECHNIQUE (supine):

1. Standing at the head of the table, place your palms on the upper chest with thumbs near the sternum and fingertips below the axilla;

2. Repetitively push the upper chest posteroinferiorly at a rate and force that causes the abdomen to move up and down, about a hundred pumps per minute;

3. Continue pumping for 1/2–2 minutes as tolerated. If effective, consider prescribing DIAPHRAGMATIC BREATHING.

4. Alternative technique:

   a) Ask the patient to take deep breaths and during exhalation repetitively pump at a rate and force that causes the abdomen to move up and down;

   b) With inhalation maintain steady compressive pressure on the upper chest;

   c) Repeat the exhalation pump and inhalation resistance for several breaths as tolerated;

   d) During the early part of the last inhalation, suddenly release hand pressure to encourage rapid lung expansion and increased venous and lymphatic return (avoid with emphysema[1]).

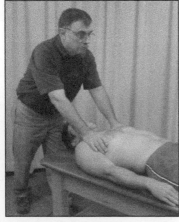

Thoracic pump

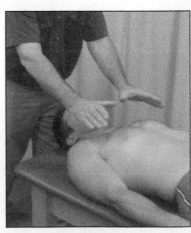

Rebound expansion

PECTORAL TRACTION

INDICATIONS: Atelectasis, bronchitis, pneumonia, peripheral edema, and other problems.

RELATIVE CONTRAINDICATIONS: Aspiration or acute rib fracture.

TECHNIQUE (supine):

1. Sit or stand at the head of the table and firmly grasp the lateral border of the pectoralis muscles at the anterior axillary folds;

2. Slowly lean backward to stretch the pectoralis muscles;

3. Ask the patient to take deep breaths and during inhalation increase pectoralis stretch, maintaining steady traction during exhalation;

4. Continue until tissue give is completed and then slowly release traction. If effective, consider prescribing DIAPHRAGMATIC BREATHING or PECTORAL STRETCH.

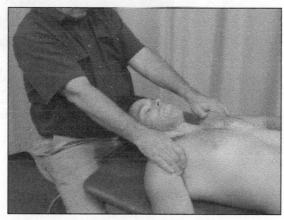

Pectoral traction

DIAPHRAGMATIC BREATHING

INDICATIONS: To improve respiration, induce relaxation response, balance autonomics; to complement thoracic pump or pectoral traction

TECHNIQUE (supine or seated):

1. Lie on your back with knees bent and a hand resting on the lower abdomen;
2. Slowly take a deep breath all the way in, allowing your abdomen to rise during inhalation;
3. Slowly let your breath all the way out, allowing the abdomen to drop during exhalation;
4. Repeat 5–10 times;
5. Do this exercise 2–4 times a day or as often as needed.

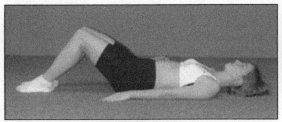

Diaphragmatic breathing

PEDAL PUMP

INDICATIONS: Peripheral edema, atelectasis, bronchitis, pneumonia, and other problems.

RELATIVE CONTRAINDICATIONS: Acute ankle sprain, acute congestive heart failure, lymphatic cancer, deep venous thrombosis, peritonitis, or recent abdominal surgery.

TECHNIQUE (supine):

1. Standing at the foot of the table, place your palms on the plantar surface of the feet with fingers over the toes;

2. Dorsiflex the feet to the restrictive barrier to stretch the fascia of the posterior compartment of the leg;

3. Repetitively lean into your palms to rhythmically dorsiflex the ankles at a rate and force that causes the abdomen to move up and down, about a hundred pumps per minute;

4. Alternative technique: Hold the dorsal surface and repetitively pull the ankles into plantar flexion;

5. Continue pumping for 1/2–2 minutes as tolerated. If effective, consider prescribing PEDAL SELF-PUMP.

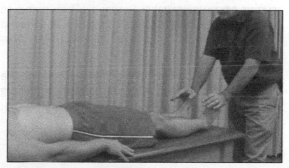

Dorsiflexion pump

PEDAL SELF-PUMP

1. Lie on your back with knees bent and toes against a wall;
2. Rapidly push your feet into the wall and release to move your abdomen up and down;
3. Repeat about twice a second for 1/2–2 minutes;
4. Do this exercise 2–4 times a day as needed.

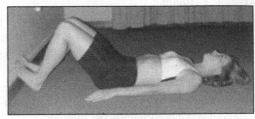

Pedal self-pump

LIVER/SPLEEN PUMP

INDICATIONS: Liver, gall bladder, or spleen dysfunction; immune stimulation (spleen pump).

RELATIVE CONTRAINDICATIONS: Peritonitis; liver pump–acute hepatitis, acute cholecystitis, undiagnosed hepatomegaly; or spleen pump—undiagnosed splenomegaly, spleen trauma, acute infectious mononucleosis.

TECHNIQUE (supine):

1. Place one hand on the costal margin overlying the involved organ and your other hand under the ribs posterior to the organ;
2. Gently compress the ribs between your hands until tissue give stops;
3. Have the patient take a deep breath, and during exhalation, repetitively compress the ribs between your hands using gentle force;
4. During early inhalation quickly release hand pressure to cause rib recoil;
5. Repeat the exhalation pump and inhalation recoil 3–5 times, if tolerated.

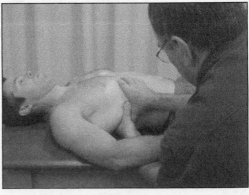

Liver pump

UPPER EXTREMITY PÉTRISSAGE

INDICATIONS: Upper extremity edema.

RELATIVE CONTRAINDICATIONS: Lymphatic or metastatic cancer, deep venous thrombosis, or compartment syndrome.

TECHNIQUE (lateral):

1. Place the patient's hand on your shoulder and interlock your fingers on the upper arm;

2. Gently squeeze the tissues and exert motion counterclockwise and clockwise toward the shoulder, repeating 3–5 times;

3. Grasp the arm above the elbow, gently squeeze the tissues, and exert motion counterclockwise and clockwise toward the shoulder, repeating 3–5 times;

4. Grasp the forearm just below the elbow, gently squeeze the tissues, and exert motion counterclockwise and clockwise toward the elbow, repeating 3–5 times;

5. Grasp the forearm just above the wrist, gently squeeze the tissues, and exert motion counterclockwise and clockwise toward the elbow, repeating 3–5 times.

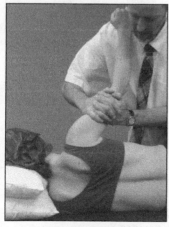

Arm pétrissage

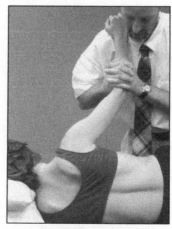

Forearm pétrissage

PISTON BREATH[2]

1. Sit upright with the arms hanging at your sides;
2. Push your shoulders backward and turn your hands outward as far as they will go, creating tension in your upper chest;
3. Breath deeply in and out through the nose using brisk but steady breaths without pause between cycles;
4. With each exhalation allow the shoulders to move farther back and the arms to turn more outward;
5. Repeat for 10 breaths, pacing yourself to avoid lightheadedness;
6. Do once a day, gradually increasing the number of breaths.

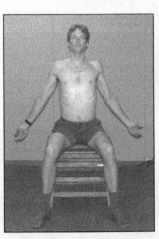

Piston breath

REFERENCES

1. Noll DR, Degenhardt BD, Johnson JC, et al. Immediate effects of osteopathic manipulative treatment in elderly patients with chronic obstructive pulmonary disease. *J Am Osteopath Assoc.* 2008;108(5):251–259.
2. Adapted from Comeaux ZC. *Robert Fulford, D.O. and the Philosopher Physician.* Seattle, WA: Eastland Press; 2002.

13 OMT in Primary Care

Osteopathic manipulative treatment (OMT) can have a major role in primary care practices in which back pain, headache, neck pain, cough, upper respiratory congestion, abdominal pain, and lower extremity problems are among the most frequent reasons for patient visits.[1] Systematic reviews have identified evidence of effectiveness of manipulation for low back pain, neck pain, and headache.[2-9] Treatment of other problems is supported by smaller studies, case reports, and clinical consensus. Meta-analyses on safety of manipulation have determined that lumbar spine treatment is relatively safe but that neck manipulation using thrust technique has a rare association with vertebral artery dissection and stroke.[10-12] It appears that other forms of cervical manipulation, such as counterstrain, myofascial release, muscle energy, and articulatory, have no such association but clinical judgment is always warranted regarding the suitability of a technique for a particular patient. Before any manipulative treatment is provided its potential benefit to the patient must be weighed against risk for that individual and availability of alternative treatments.

Integration of OMT into a busy practice requires examination and treatment skills that are both efficacious and time efficient. Skillful observation for asymmetry, palpation for tension and tenderness, and range of motion testing can facilitate patient evaluation, refining both differential diagnosis and diagnostic testing. Treatment models that have been successful at streamlining osteopathic diagnosis and treatment for primary care practices include regional assessment, identification of key somatic dysfunction, fascial diaphragm evaluation and treatment, pediatric application of osteopathy in the cranial field, and integration of different techniques.

The **region of complaint** is the first cue many osteopathic physicians use to determine if somatic dysfunction is significantly related to symptoms. Although it is always desirable to evaluate beyond just the area of complaint to screen for additional or contributing somatic dysfunction, this may not always be possible in a busy primary care setting. Therefore, it is useful to be able to efficiently diagnose and treat the key lesion in a region. Screening tests presented in each region chapter can be used to quickly assess for the presence or absence of somatic dysfunction related to the chief complaint. The absence of somatic dysfunction or persistence of symptoms after an initial treatment indicates a need to evaluate regions on either side (front/back, above/below, or left/right) of the region of chief complaint. Chronic problems often require more detailed examination for systemic, postural, or multifactorial problems, including consideration of visceral and mind–body–spiritual influences.

315

Chronic low back pain has been associated with six key somatic dysfunctions termed the **dirty half dozen**[13]

1. Nonneutral lumbar (single segment);

2. Pubic compression or shear;

3. Extended sacrum (backward torsion or unilateral extension);

4. Innominate shear (downslip, upslip, and unilateral sacral flexion);

5. Short leg/sacral base unleveling;

6. Muscle imbalance of trunk or lower extremities.

Evaluation for these causes of chronic low back pain can be achieved by selected palpation and motion testing. Landmarks for palpation include standing iliac crest height, medial malleolus, anterior superior iliac spine, pubic symphysis, posterior superior iliac spine, sacral base and inferior lateral angle, lumbar transverse processes, and tender points for iliacus, piriformis, and iliolumbar ligaments. Motion testing for sacroiliac joints, sacrum, and lumbar spine completes the diagnosis. Treatment of the identified cause with OMT, flexibility exercises, and postural retraining can help some people afflicted with failed low back syndrome. In some cases, evaluation of the lower thoracic spine, ribs, or even more remote regions can identify an additional cause of chronic low back pain.

Upper back pain can be efficiently evaluated by palpatory screening for **single segment** and **key rib** somatic dysfunctions. Paravertebral fullness, spasm, or rotation restriction at a single vertebral level is more often causative of pain than group somatic dysfunctions. Treatment of a single segment restriction (type 2, nonneutral) will often resolve surrounding group dysfunctions. The role of the cervical spine and upper extremities should also be considered in the clinical evaluation.

Chronic headache has been related to **cervical and nonphysiological head somatic dysfunctions**. Persistent occipitoatlantal, atlantoaxial, and typical cervical joint restrictions can be treated to help some people with chronic tension headaches. Sphenobasilar compressions, vertical strains, or lateral strains are diagnosed by palpation of sphenoid greater wings and occiput during cranial flexion and extension. Treatment of these cranial base somatic dysfunctions can be achieved with sphenobasilar compression–decompression or balanced membranous tension techniques. In resistant cases of chronic headache, it is useful to also evaluate the temporomandibular joint, trapezius muscle, upper to mid-thoracic spine, and sacrum.

Chest wall pain is frequently associated with a **key rib** somatic dysfunction. The key rib, when treated, resolves other rib tender points or motion restrictions. Rib somatic dysfunctions linked to a key rib include

Inhalation group—inferior rib;
Exhalation group—superior rib;

Multiple rib tender points—anterior or posterior subluxed rib;
Bilateral rib somatic dysfunction—corresponding thoracic vertebra

Treatment of a related thoracic dysfunction may resolve rib somatic dysfunction. If not, treatment of the key rib instead of all ribs can significantly reduce treatment time. It is useful to also evaluate the sternum and diaphragm in resistant or recurrent cases.

Key lesion screening can be used to quickly identify the most clinically significant region of somatic dysfunction. Motion is induced or palpated on alternating sides of the body and the resultant vector of tension usually points to the region of most significant restriction. Examples of key lesion screening include LOWER EXTREMITY DIAGNOSIS USING INHERENT MOTION, PELVIS DIAGNOSIS USING INHERENT MOTION, SACRAL DIAGNOSIS USING INHERENT MOTION, THORACIC/RIB DIAGNOSIS USING INHERENT MOTION, ACROMION DROP TEST, THORACIC INLET DIAGNOSIS USING INHERENT MOTION, KEY LESION SCREENING USING EXTREMITIES, and KEY LESION SCREENING USING COMPRESSION. Once identified, the region of most significant restriction can receive more specific examination as well as treatment using the appropriate principles outlined in Chapter 1.

Multiregion or systemic dysfunctions can be efficiently diagnosed and treated using **fascial patterns**.[14] Four transverse fascial diaphragms can be quickly tested with the patient supine and categorized as ideal (no restriction), compensated (alternating restrictions), or uncompensated (not alternating). The fascial diaphragms and their corresponding fascial exam and vertebrae are

1. Pelvic diaphragm—lumbosacral fascia—L5–S1;
2. Thoracic diaphragm—thoracolumbar fascia—T12–L3;
3. Thoracic inlet—cervicothoracic fascia—C7–T4;
4. Foramen magnum—occipitoatlantal fascia—OA–C2.

Treatment of the uncompensated or restricted fascial diaphragms or corresponding vertebral segments can improve overall postural compensation, lymphatic drainage, and recovery from illness. For a patient with pneumonia, treating the diaphragm and thoracic inlet facilitates the effectiveness of rib raising and thoracic pump at improving respiration and lung drainage. Release of tension in the thoracic inlet is important for any lymphatic treatment because the thoracic duct passes through Sibson fascia twice on its course to the subclavian vein (see THORACIC DUCT

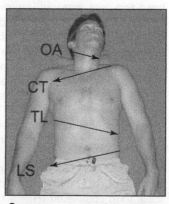

Common compensatory pattern

IN THORACIC INLET). Treating the pelvic and thoracic diaphragms of a patient with constipation or paralytic ileus improves the ability of thoracolumbar inhibition and mesenteric lift to promote peristalsis.

THORACIC DUCT IN THORACIC INLET

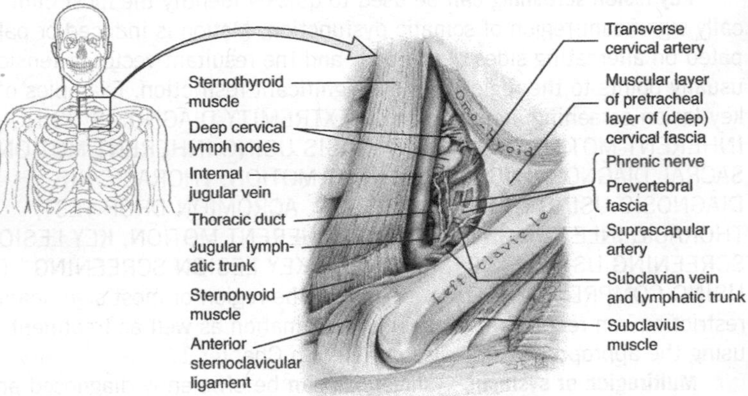

Transverse cervical artery
Muscular layer of pretracheal layer of (deep) cervical fascia
Phrenic nerve
Prevertebral fascia
Suprascapular artery
Subclavian vein and lymphatic trunk
Subclavius muscle
Sternothyroid muscle
Deep cervical lymph nodes
Internal jugular vein
Thoracic duct
Jugular lymphatic trunk
Sternohyoid muscle
Anterior sternoclavicular ligament
Omohyoid
Left clavicle
Anterior view

Lymph flows superiorly through Sibson fascia before descending into subclavian vein

Several common **pediatric conditions** can sometimes be helped with the addition of osteopathic treatment. **Recurrent acute otitis media** in children is due, in part, to impaired functioning of the eustachian tube leading to fluid retention in the middle ear. When the eustachian tube is not draining properly fluid accumulates in the middle ear leading to recurrent infection and hearing problems. Osteopathic treatment of the head and neck area can improve drainage of the middle ear and thereby reduce recurrent infections and secondary hearing impairment (see MANDIBULAR DRAINAGE). **Infantile colic** is frequently associated with compression of the base of the skull. This is presumed to lead to a compression neuropathy of the vagus nerve, thereby leading to autonomic dysregulation of gastrointestinal activity and colic. Gentle decompression of this area allows establishment of normal bowel function and relief from the colic (see OCCIPITAL DECOMPRESSION).

Experienced practitioners often **integrate two or more techniques** for a more efficient treatment. For example, a patient with piriformis syndrome causing sciatic neuritis might initially be positioned for PIRIFORMIS COUNTERSTRAIN but, instead of holding the patient in the position of relief for 90 seconds, the doctor might follow any tissue release until completed (HIP MYOFASCIAL RELEASE) and then move the hip into its internal rotation restriction, asking the patient to push away against resistance before moving to a new restrictive barrier (HIP MUSCLE ENERGY). Treatment of someone with lateral epicondylitis might begin with ELBOW MYOFASCIAL RELEASE and then move into FOREARM MUSCLE ENERGY before applying a RADIAL HEAD THRUST, all done in one continuous motion. This integration of techniques is very effective when based on the somatic dysfunction and its initial response to treatment.

Although the primary care application of osteopathic diagnosis and treatment distinguishes osteopathic medicine, even more important is the underlying philosophy that guides the use of these skills. In the words of Marlene A. Wager, DO, Emeritus Professor of Family Medicine at WVSOM:

"The philosophy of treating the body as a whole, the holistic approach to patients, the knowledge that the body can heal itself, especially if in true alignment which can be accomplished by manipulation of the musculoskeletal system . . . this is osteopathic medicine."

REFERENCES

1. American Academy of Family Physicians. Facts about family practice, 2005. Available at: http://www.aafp.org/x530.xml
2. Bronfort G, Assendelft WJ, Evans R, et al. Efficacy of spinal manipulation for chronic headache: a systematic review. *J Manipulative Physiol Ther*. 2001; 24(7):457–466.
3. Bronfort G, Haas M, Evans R, et al. Efficacy of spinal manipulation and mobilization for low back pain and neck pain: a systematic review and best evidence synthesis. *Spine J*. 2004;4(3):335–356.
4. Gross AR, Hoving JL, Haines TA, et al. A Cochrane review of manipulation and mobilization for mechanical neck disorders. *Spine*. 2004;15(29): 1541–1548.
5. Gross AR, Kay T, Hondras M, et al. Manual therapy for mechanical neck disorders: a systematic review. *Man Ther*. 2002;7(3):131–149.
6. Hurwitz EL, Aker PD, Adams AH, et al. Manipulation and mobilization of the cervical spine: a systematic review of the literature. *Spine*. 1996;21(15):1746–1759.
7. Koes BW, Assendelft WJ, Van der Heijden G, et al. Spinal manipulation for low back pain: an updated systematic review of randomized clinical trials. *Spine*. 1996;21(24):2860–2871.
8. Pengel HM. Systematic review of conservative interventions for subacute low back pain. *Clin Rehabil*. 2002;16(8):811–820.
9. van Tulder MW, Koes BW, Bouter LM. Conservative treatment of acute and chronic nonspecific low back pain: a systematic review of randomized controlled trials of the most common interventions. *Spine*. 1997;22(18): 2128–2156.
10. Oliphant D. Safety of spinal manipulation in the treatment of lumbar disc herniations: a systematic review and risk assessment. *J Manipulative Physiol Ther*. 2004;27(3):197–210.

11. Rubinstein SM, Peerdeman SM, van Tulder MW, et al. A systematic review of the risk factors for cervical artery dissection. *Stroke*. 2005;36(7):1575–1580.
12. Stevinson C, Ernst E. Risks associated with spinal manipulation. *Am J Med*. 2002;112(7):566–571.
13. Greenman PE. *Principles of Manual Medicine*. 2nd ed. Baltimore, MD: Williams & Wilkins; 1996.
14. Kuchera ML, Kappler RE. Clinical significance of fascial patterns. In: Ward RC, ed. *Foundations for Osteopathic Medicine*. 2nd ed. Philadelphia, PA: Lippincott Williams & Wilkins; 2003:583–584.

INDEX

Note: Page numbers followed by f and t indicate figures and tables, respectively.